Praise for John Blade and *Pandemic Armor*

"This is a thoughtful book, loaded with some of the most important lessons and advice to be discovered to improve your wellbeing. Let the ideas inspire you to take control over your immunity!"

Brian Tracy
author, speaker, and consultant

PANDEMIC
A·R·M·O·R
MAXIMUM
IMMUNITY

PANDEMIC A·R·M·O·R

MAXIMUM IMMUNITY

JOHN BLADE
OTRL, CFT/CPT, CAPS, ACLS

Book design and artwork by G Sharp Design, LLC.
www.gsharpmajor.com

ISBN# 979-8-88502-011-4 (e-book)
ISBN# 979-8-88502-012-1 (audiobook)
ISBN# 979-8-88502-013-8 (paperback)
ISBN# 979-8-88502-014-5 (hardcover)

Library of Congress Control Number: 2022903647

Pandemic Armor has been filed for copyright.

Other Books by John Blade

EXERLEAN

Total Body Fat Incinerator

Weight Chaining

CONTENTS

BRIEF

infection: the state produced by the establishment of one or more pathogenic agents (such as bacteria, protozoans, or viruses) in or on the body of a suitable host (*Merriam-Webster*)

host: a living animal or plant on or in which a parasite lives (*Merriam-Webster*)

portal of entry: how a pathogen enters a susceptible host (Centers for Disease Control and Prevention)

INTRODUCTION

You are either immune or susceptible to sickness, disease, and death. In times of a pandemic, plague, or communal illness, the susceptible die, and the immune survive. It is imperative that you maximize your immunity and establish pandemic armor. To do this, you may need to abandon some of the blatant characteristics, behaviors, and traits of the susceptible you are harboring.

In this book, you will learn who dies and who lives during a global pandemic. You will learn how to shed the traits of susceptibility and replace them with those of maximum immunity. Don't become a statistic of disability or death by taking an about-face to the situation. Your time to act is now. Millions die each year due to viruses, infections, and diseases. You don't have to be one of them.

The human body is a miraculous machine with internal mechanisms that can keep you young or age you with haste, make you healthier or sicker, or make you slower or faster. What you do, eat, think, and speak determines your level of immunity to viruses, pandemic killers, and the negative Nancys who will forever attempt to keep you down, attempt to stop your progress, and sabotage your mission to change yourself for the better. Yeah, there are worse things than viruses. Negative people.

It is time to enter the unimaginable realms of the COVID-19 front-lines and uncover the truth about who dies and who lives, to reveal insider information on why living after infection may not mean you're in the clear. Many who survive the COVID-19 frontlines continue living with a grave disability. I want to take you on a journey of self-discovery, new learning, and awareness. Let's embark on a mission to learn and earn your pandemic armor, thus donning maximum immunity.

SECTION ONE
THE PATHOGEN

CHAPTER ONE
THE PRONE TEAM

Pancakes are abundant in here. But a drizzle of delicious syrup, a smidgen of melted butter, and a dusting of powdered sugar are not on the menu. These flapjacks are instead coated with copious mucus and crusty snot, with smeared or pooled bowel. They are constantly saturated in urine, not syrup. And they are generously sprinkled with baby powder on top of lathered salve.

These are not pancakes but real people. Most are intubated with a plastic tube strategically placed down their throats so as not to inflate the stomach but the lungs. The mechanical ventilator breathes for them. Some have urine catheters, some have rectal tubes, and most have a tree of IV bags previously unseen in my twenty-plus years working in the hospital setting. These are the COVID-19 patients who are being proned. Most display oddly dispersed bruising, bloated faces, and lips so swollen collagen implants dim in comparison. I cannot imagine a person being in a less demeaning and immodest situation.

They nonetheless lie unaware.

Unaware that death weighs heavy on the scale of odds.

They would already be dead without this burdening process. This is their last hope.

We are their last hope.

In the hospital bed, they lie strewn out in the nude, affixed with tape pasties to protect their nipples—males and females—to prevent them from shearing off during the rotations or sustaining tissue decay from prolonged pressure. Too much time in one position can lead to skin and underlying tissue death due to lack of circulation—suffocation of the cells, you might say. This is why we prone. These people appear departed as we flip one after another down the COVID-19 frontline.

Supine to prone, prone to supine, three to four times a day, this is the way.

Proning is to place a human facedown; to place them faceup is supining. Proning or supining an intubated or nonintubated COVID-19 patient involves rotating them like a marshmallow on a stick. You've got to be careful not to leave it in one spot too long or it might turn brown, then burn, and soon after light up in flames before quickly disintegrating. And continuing with our analogy, leaving skin under pressure is like leaving a marshmallow in the flame too long. First is the formation of a supple area, then an opening in the skin, which left unattended will lead to ulcers. These deepening craters extend through the skin to fat, muscle, and even bone. Eventually necrosis or infection or both set in, and in the worst-case scenario—which is not death, at least not yet—amputation is required.

Other than relieving pressure, proning also uses the power of gravity to help mobilize fluids in the lungs. It's like a sponge in a water bucket—it cannot release the water by sitting inside the bucket, but if you lift it out and give it a good squeezing, the water falls out of the sponge. But we cannot squeeze a human being. We can only reposition them, hoping that gravity will move fluids and help the patient regain respiratory function. In some circumstances, the doctor can perform a thoracentesis—stabbing a long straight needle into a waterlogged lung cavity and drawing out the smothering liquid, giving the patient instant relief.

Like fluid in the lungs, blood in the circulatory system has mass and weight, so it is also pulled toward the earth by gravity. A beating heart is all that stops the blood in your body from pooling to the dependent side—the downside. That's your feet if you're standing, your backside if you're supine, or your frontside if you're prone. At rest, the heart slows, the force of circulation is low, and the need for repositioning is vital. This is why we roll. If a person cannot reposition themselves, their blood will pool, coagulate, and clot. If clots form, they can travel through the bloodstream and lead to a stroke in the brain, cause emboli in the lungs, or stop blood flow to an external appendage. Say hello to high risk of amputation, disability, and death. Now add to this dilemma an even greater risk of clotting due to COVID-19. Using a power-adjustable hospital bed and the proning protocol, we can rotate, tilt, roll, and pillow-up a person. The result is pressure relief, fluid mobilization, and clot and pneumonia prevention.

Rotating a patient like a marshmallow may not be the best representation of proning, as a marshmallow is almost weightless while the COVID patient, usually obese, is of unfathomable dead weight. The proning process is more like rolling over a dead bear. The process to prone a patient takes at least eight staff members, each wearing a biohazard negative pressure respirator or N95 mask with a surgical mask layered over it, an eye shield, a yellow droplet gown, a hair guard, and double gloves. I am denied the use of an N95 mask because I refuse to shave off the goatee I have owned for over twenty-seven years. Shaving this off would be like cutting off my left testicle. So I am left with wearing a respirator hood called a powered air-purifying respirator (PAPR), or "papper" for short.

If you could be present to observe me proning, you might think I am one of those biohazard or hazmat characters in a virus movie. *Vroooom* goes the respirator as I depress the button for the start-up sequence. My biohazard hood blows up, and little holes allow the air to escape. This negative pressure suit sucks air in and filters it, then pressure pushes it out. The PAPR is old and reusable; the plastic front shields are a little blurry from years' worth of scratches, and it sounds like a vacuum is going at my ear. No contaminated air from outside the hood is allowed in because the incoming filtered air is continuously pushed out. The other option, a controlled air-purifying respirator (CAPR), "or capper," is only available for doctors and nurses, not mealy therapists unless you got lucky and fitted before the first COVID surge. This is the third surge.

Yelling at each other to hear, we mentally prepare to enter the infectious room. We are desperate not to get this disease, and being healthcare workers on the frontline, our risk is high. Fear of getting it is the unspoken underlying truth we endure in this hell on earth.

* * *

Before standing at the doors to purgatory, my alarm sang its digital song at precisely 3:00 a.m. When I wake up, I wake up. No snooze button or thinking in bed after the alarm goes off. "Get up when you wake up," says Bob Proctor. In agreement, I swiftly put my feet on the floor, head to the kitchen's supplement zone, slam some caffeinated pre-workout aminos, and then venture to my home gym to jam out forty-five minutes on the elliptical while reading *The New Earth* by Eckhart Tolle. I'm trying to stay centered during this pandemic. I am preparing my mind and body for the day—maximizing my immunity before entering the COVID inferno.

After cardio and reading, I write from 4:00 a.m. to 5:00 a.m. Since the beginning of this pandemic, I have witnessed the devastating effects of a COVID-19 infection. After discovering that all the predominant traits are preventable, I felt a deep desire to help people prevent this kind of susceptibility to disease and sickness and took it upon myself to write this book.

I am in the trenches of the COVID-19 pandemic going on twenty months now. I have expertise in rehabilitation, fitness, bodybuilding, dieting, health, and wellness. I am a board-certified and licensed occupational therapist (OT), a certified personal trainer (CPT) and National Physique Committee (NPC) bodybuilding athlete, and a Certified Aging-in-Place Specialist (CAPS). I am by design destined to help people transform their body composition and lifestyle for the better. I am bold, deliberate, and passionate about this. That's why the preventable nature of low immunity in most COVID-19 patients weighs heavy on my heart.

At 6:00 a.m., I start my eight to ten hours of work as a full-time OT in an acute care hospital. I see eight to fourteen patients a day depending on whether I can attain a flow state. Otherwise, I will persevere as best I can through the wavy waters of the hospital pandemic chaos. I have seen thousands and thousands of patients over the last two decades— long enough to know there are obvious trends for those admitted to hospitals. The observable and objective evidence is clear that certain behaviors, traits, actions, inactions, habits, genetics, and body compositions will inevitably admit you to a hospital someday. And these causes are mostly *preventable*. The chances of seeing a healthy, lean, and athletic person admitted to the hospital are near zero, no matter the age. I have observed thousands of patients desperately and miserably trying to stay alive on COVID row. None of these affected patients are lean, none are healthy, and all have preventable comorbidities.

The winter mornings of the COVID-19 2020, 2021, and 2022 pandemic are dark, dry, and cold as a yeti's tit. My truck sits outside coated in ice because our garage looks like we're hoarders. After scraping the windows, warming up the motor, and securing my homemade duct tape and cardboard man purse, it is time to go. Driving to work, I prepare my mind for what is coming. I pray to God for the wisdom and strength to help my patients and at the end of the day return home without a lifting injury, shit on my shoes, or a new disease.

Before exiting my truck in the parking garage, I don my mask and place my lanyard around my neck so that when I get to the double doors, I can badge myself in. See, we are in lockdown. Doors that were once open to the public 24/7 are now secured. As I walk through the doors, I haven't entered the gates of hell yet. No, those are coming. I walk the purgatorial halls of the outer rim of the hospital with the realization that there is no turning back. The frontline experience is coming.

From the double doors, down the outer rim, I arrive at the rehab department. This is home base for me, a therapist. From here I clock in, take my temperature and document in the log, sanitize my hands, sit down to my computer, and prepare my patient list. Next, I grab a set of nursing scrubs and put them on. I am preparing to prone.

Outside the COVID cohort—the infection zone—are PAPRs, scrubs, eye shields, nursing scrubs, sanitization wipes, hair covers, and hundreds of manila envelopes stored in plastic tubs all down the hallway. Each envelope has an employee's name on it and holds their N95 mask and biohazard gear.

During the first surge, back in March 2020, we had to reuse our disposable surgical masks for days except for the lucky few assigned N95 masks. I had to bring my own N95 from home before hospital-wide guidance allowed this, and approving it took three visits and a sit-down with the upper echelon. "It will just be giving you a false sense of security," they told me. *Yeah, right, tell that to Dr. Fauci,* I said to myself. We are soldiers fighting in the war to help patients survive, all the while desperately trying to prevent getting infected ourselves. We are in a war against this virus in ways nobody outside healthcare can understand.

Eleven months later, in winter 2020, we could change to a new paper mask daily—but not like before, still not between patients. The same went for eye shields and N95 masks. We had been trained for eons to dispose of this contaminated personal protective equipment when leaving the infected or a potentially infectious patient room. Nope, not during a pandemic. Supplies like PPE are running short at all times. We must preserve.

The Frontline

The designated prone team scrubs are light, fit comfortably, and match my blue eyes. My Hokas are mine—they're not disposable shoes. I've tried many brands of shoes over the years, and these are the only ones that prevent the aching that occurs from walking on concrete hospital floors ten hours a day. They are gold. They are valued. I need to make sure that when I leave the cohort, I wipe down and saturate them with virus-killing liquid and, please God, don't allow feces or urine to land on them today. I have had to discard a few pairs of expensive shoes due to loose stooling falling on my shoes as I help the patients out of bed. This is a minor issue that comes with the job of being a hospital therapist. Shit, piss, snot, puss, and contagion. It's everywhere.

Being distressed by the possibility of bringing COVID-19 home to my wife and three kids is a constant. Not happening—not on my watch.

I wash my hands a hundred or more times a day and bathe them—and sometimes my forearms, head, neck, and face—in alcohol foam. It's total overkill—or maybe not. Nobody knows the truth. I follow all necessary and over-the-top preventable measures. This is my life, not theirs.

After donning my scrubs, the PAPR belt and respirator pump are strapped tight to my waist and the biohazard hood is draped forward over my right shoulder. Now it is time to go through the pristine white gates to hell. The COVID cohort. The frontline. The contamination zone. The place of the living dead. The place of the not dead but appear to be dead, may be dead soon, or may be zombies. *Is there contagion on the nickel-plated door handle—on my hand? Where is the sanitizing hand foam?* We're all in the same hell with the same worries, stress, burnout, and pain. Once on the frontline, all I can see is station after station of precaution carts placed evenly down the long corridor, each loaded with all the paraphernalia that will protect us from the virus. The stench of the necromancer's breath lingers in the air—or is that still shit, piss, and mysterious body fluids? Maybe the grim reaper is taking a dump. There aren't many options to cover up the stench of sickness and plague—maybe the anosmia (loss of smell) that COVID causes is a good thing here since it forces you to breathe through your mouth.

Straining to see through the hazy PAPR eye shield, it is difficult to recognize anyone. We all look the same. Yellow contact precautions gowns over blue scrubs, PAPRs and CAPRs, N95 masks, surgical masks, rubber gloves, and the essence of death—the humming of a vacuum factory in the backdrop. Nurses are scurrying here and there, working their butts off caring for the never-ending demands of a COVID patient.

There's the prone team, I think as I finally catch a glimpse of someone preparing to flip pancakes. This environment is so depressing we must make light of it to preserve our sanity and decompress the madness.

"Ready to do this, guys?" Another department boss volunteers for this position.

I don't. I am assigned. Do it or die.

She is the bomb. Anyone who volunteers for this and has the kind of vigor she does is a pandemic enigma—a great leader in times of fear and the unknown.

The prone team of eight enters the patient room and quickly shuts the door behind them so as not to let the virus out of the room. As if it isn't already out, but just in case, we must prevent escape. Eight fully geared-up staff members and a COVID patient. One of us is a respiratory therapist, an RT, or an anesthesiologist. The RT or anesthesiologist manages the patient's head and ventilator during the proning process. Their job is to make sure the ventilator tube doesn't pull out and that we don't twist the patient's head off. Another member, usually the patient's primary RN, manages the multitude of IV lines, tube feedings, and ICU (intensive care unit) monitoring devices. Three of us line up on each side of the patient's bed, the RT or anesthesiologist stands at the head of the bed, and the eighth person stands at the foot of the bed to call out the steps of the proning process. This is to make sure we all are on the same page during the flip. Sometimes an extra nurse or nursing assistant manages the patient's bed padding, cleanup of stool and urine incontinence, skin inspection, and other necessary tasks of patient care.

Bedsheet, incontinence pad, and slip sheet wrap both sides of the patient hoagie. Whether the patient is supine or prone, the flip always occurs in one rotation in the same direction, toward the ventilator. First, the staff on each side roll up the many layers of bedding. Then when the leader calls out to flip, like synchronous swimmers in harmonious motion, we rotate the patient on their side, scoot them a few inches toward the side of the bed, and finally place them on the opposite side of where they were.

In one proning, I witnessed a staff member on the other side accidentally catch his thumb on the bottom of his CAPR, causing it to flip off his chin during the rotation and pop off his face, exposing him to the contagious environment. With a "holy shit" look on his face, he frantically returned his mask to its protective position. Healthcare workers must be—have to be—in the riskiest position for infection on this planet. We are essential.

After tidying up the patient and their bedding and making sure we are no longer needed, the prone team goes through the decontamination process before exiting the room. We head to the next infected room, hit the cart outside for a new set of double gloves, pause to breathe in, exhale, and prep to do the same process all over again, until all the necessary patients have been proned. When we are all finished, we disinfect the PAPRs and CAPRs, place our N95 masks and eye shields back in our manila envelopes, put our scrubs in the dirty utility bin, don our clean clothes, and—for me—go back to my real job as an occupational therapist, to get all the regular patients out of bed and moving. Sometimes, before I hit the hospital floor with the non-COVID patients, I start to worry that I missed a spot during decontamination, so I wipe everything down again, just to make sure. Then in eight hours, the prone team meets to do it all again.

Based on COVID admissions to our hospital, you have at least a 9.2 percent chance of death if admitted for COVID, a 31.6 percent chance if in the ICU for COVID, and over a 90 percent chance of death if intubated with COVID. Those who are infected yet not hospitalized are much better off, with less debility and a much lower death rate. Some have no effects of COVID at all. The asymptomatic are the people *out there*, not *in the hospital*, mostly kids, teens, young adults, the lean, athletic, and healthy. Some may experience a tinge of flu-like or cold-like symptoms, and others nothing at all.

There exist polarizing paradigms of people. The maskers and the antimaskers. The seeing firsthand—that is, the frontline healthcare workers—and everyone else outside of the hospital frontline, who know only what the government officials, the CDC, the WHO, social media, and the news media tell them. All different messages, messages of facts from credible and trusted sources surrounded by an ocean of fearmongering, misinformation, and delusional theories of political power, government conspiracy, the mark of the beast, and the end of days. Like that colorful and weathered homeless woman on the corner waving her "the end is near!" sign, these prophecies, thousands of them over thousands of years, have all proven false. A pandemic presents the perfect environment for new revelations and prophecies, new paranoia and fear, radical ideation, and mayhem. The truth is lost in all the noise and chaos. All of us as therapists, doctors, and other frontline workers are learning as we go, and we are desperately trying to avoid the delusions of crowds—the conspiracy theories, mass hysteria, and psychological chaos that can develop during unusually stressful events, which consequently negatively affect the population as a whole.

Whether a person believes COVID-19 is real or not, a worldwide pandemic is here. We have no choice in the matter. It is affecting all of us in one way or another.

Most don't see what I see as a healthcare worker on the frontlines of this pandemic.

But I see what they see, too, because a frontline worker like me does have a normal life outside of work. I understand how it can be difficult to comprehend the anxiety about "the surge."

From my position, it is much easier to see through the chaos . . . to understand both sides of the line. I am in the middle. I see the worst-case scenario of this pandemic in the hospital. I see the debilitating effects of this virus, the disability, the dying, and the survivors—the living dead. From outside the hospital, nobody can see the coronavirus, or the desperately sick people, or the overburdened healthcare system, or the healthcare workers who were burnt out almost two years ago, yet still endure the burn. I am witnessing a new form of posttraumatic stress disorder (PTSD) developing—specific to healthcare workers and others working the frontlines during a pandemic. I don't know what else to call it—the horrible stuff we see, the risk we place ourselves in all day long every day, the fear of sickness, death, or worse yet, being the contagious pathway between COVID and our loved ones.

There is no way to predict the future, but I feel, based on what is taking place in the hospital environment right now, that it is highly possible there is going to be a mass exodus of healthcare workers in the near future. If there is, it will be mainly due to an already underlying developing issue—the exponentially rising percentage of obese patients and the sheer physical difficulty of taking care of these people. Obese patients are unintentionally disabling healthcare workers with spine, hip, knee, shoulder, ankle, and hand injuries at an ascending rate. The laborious healthcare burden of the bariatric patient (*bariatric* is the medical term for everything related to being heavy or obese, such as requiring heavy-duty equipment) is surmounting natural human caregiver capability, and there is no relief in sight. Patients just keep getting fatter and fatter, and with fatter comes sicker and sicker, until they're disposed to making the hospital their new home.

Almost every single admitted COVID patient is deconditioned, sedentary, and obese or morbidly obese. The frontline looks more like an obesity pandemic than anything else. This pandemic may be just the tipping point. The tipping point for the heavy lifters in healthcare to make a change in scenery, retire, or change their career paradigm completely. Everyone has a breaking point.

The dawn of the Obesiboomers is here. The flood of fat people is upon us.

Ticktock, ticktock.

Are you one of them?

The Flip Side: Pre-vaccine Rollout

The 2020 winter from hell surges into unknown chaos. They talk about a COVID-19 vaccine, but at this time, it is just talk. No person has been vaccinated yet, and until vaccination of the flock takes place, the lightness of peace is difficult to feel. I never thought—none of us thought—that we would have to experience firsthand an active plague or live through a real worldwide viral torment. Now we all know the reality of living in a time of an unrestricted coronavirus, a pandemic.

Damn this contagious unseen hell on earth—this microscopic muthafucka is putting an unimaginable kink in our lives, disabling some and killing the rest. This is the shit we watch in sci-fi and horror movies or have read about in history books. Experiencing it firsthand is something else—please, God, bring an end to this.

The gyms are empty, and we are getting fatter. The fat are getting fatter. Kids have lost a large chunk of their needed childhood socialization, education, and typical schooling experiences. That is, if you consider the short life span of early, adolescent, and teen development. What will the consequences be from lost socialization, lost education, excess sedentary time binge-watching TV, and prolonged vegetating in the depths of the internet of things? We may never know.

Many of us wish we would have been better prepared for this. In better physical health for this. But other than having been stocked up ahead of time on extra toilet paper, paper towels, N95 masks, Sani-Wipes, meat, guns, and ammunition, almost everything is out of our control.

The only thing that matters, outside of all the noise, is whether or not the pathogen kills you or somebody you love. If you're admitted to the hospital with COVID and survive the virus, will you end up one of the undead—a zombie?

CHAPTER TWO
THE ZOMBIES

"Weeding out the herd" is a common saying that refers to the events of mother nature thinning a herd for survival of the herd as a whole. When the herd is thinned, it is the weak, slow, old, and sick who are thinned from the herd first. Predators play an important part in fulfilling this process. Predators hunt, kill, and consume the slowest, oldest, weakest, and inattentive of species. This is one aspect of the harmonious balance for all life. The wounded sheep is the first to grab the attention of the hungry wolf. Being drawn toward the path of least resistance is instinctual in all life-forms, including humans. But humans are different in that we can consciously and unconsciously think and, with intelligence beyond known reason, divert from instinct, choose a path regardless of level of difficulty, and seek to kill the strongest in the herd. We desire to eat the strong, healthy goat, not the sick, young, or weak one. We are the apex predator on this planet.

Or are some of us weeds?

Pandemics are one way to filter the weeds from the healthy plants. And they are not new.

The history of mankind shows us that pathogens may be our greatest predator. For we are the host at the mercy of the parasite.

Many of the greatest civilizations in history have fallen apart sequentially after a terrible pandemic. Take for instance the fall of Rome in AD 476—reduced from an empire of over one million to a surviving twenty thousand. That is a high death rate. The massive loss of life post-pandemic is due not just to pandemic deaths but also the subsequent economic fallout, wars and other broadscale conflicts, crime, and other sickness that were ultimately a consequence or spin-off of the pandemic. Pandemics can therefore be considered a natural phenomenon that weeds out the herd.

Rome expanded into the great Byzantine Empire only to be chipped away at by invading barbarians—the Germanic tribes. This went on for centuries. Meanwhile, the Romans were dealing with intermittent plagues. The Justinianic plague, otherwise known as the bubonic plague, was a pandemic that killed up to one hundred million people between multiple recurrences over a couple hundred years. This same pathogen was responsible for the Black Death, which is estimated to have later killed one-third to one-half of all Europeans between 1347 and 1351.

During the Black Death pandemic, a story from the memoir of the Italian Gabriele de'Mussi depicts possibly the first use of biological warfare. In the fourteenth century, the city of Caffa in Crimea was attacked by the Mongols. Hill-high piles of plague-infected cadavers were launched into the city with catapults, instilling the stench of hell and the pathogen of Black Death to its residents. Escaping survivors spread the disease to the outer realms of the Mediterranean.

Hitting closest to home is the Spanish flu of 1918, the most catastrophic pandemic before COVID-19. As many as fifty million people of all ages worldwide are believed to have died from the Spanish flu. It followed a similar course to COVID. Simultaneous to World War I, small surges in the spring were followed by more surges in the summer.

Overcrowding and the global movement of troops helped spread the virus, and in October of the same year, the surge of all surges hit. With a severe shortage of nurses, nearly two hundred thousand Americans died in that month alone. A third surge hit in early 1919, and by the spring, the Spanish flu was nearly eradicated. Maybe, just maybe, pathogens are destined to thin the herd of the sick, the weak, those with comorbidities, and those otherwise susceptible . . . those without pandemic armor.

The years of COVID-19 have been filled with bouts of mandatory isolation, business shutdowns, mask restrictions, social distancing, easing of restrictions, and a return to indoor dining. Underneath the chaos, we are all aware that at some point in the future, these restrictions and adjustments will all be gone. How many will die in the meantime before we're all vaccinated, though, or will COVID fizzle out and eventually die? How many times will the SARS-CoV-2 virus mutate and introduce variants with elevated resistance? The R.1, Alpha, Beta, Gamma, Epsilon, Theta, Zeta, Delta, Mu, and Omicron variants delivered rising resistance to human immunity. What's next? Will COVID mutate so many times that it finally delivers the "Thanos" variant . . . the End Game? That is the question we ponder as healthcare workers.

As I write this book, we continue to live in the unknown. Will the shutdown of business, social distancing, social isolation, quarantines, and masking halt a potential massive surge, the likes of which took place in the death surge of the Spanish flu? We hope so. Would herd immunity with no restrictions have been a better path, allowing the virus to take its natural course of transmission and infection until it was no longer deadly? Or will the waves of strict social distancing, mask mandates, online schooling, and business shutdowns slow the spread of COVID-19 so well that the virus has time to mutate into worse versions over and over again until it morphs into something so transmissible that it's apocalyptically deadly? We hope not.

Zombies refers to those admitted to the hospital with COVID and survive but with lingering health consequences. The living dead, we call them. Many of them are not the same as before, and they may never be. Many leave in a wheelchair, disabled and susceptible to returning to the hospital. Even the seemingly unaffected who are not admitted to a hospital complain of the lingering effects of COVID months after infection. What has the coronavirus done to our insides—our blood, our organs, and our immunity? The unknown may become apparent in the years to come, but this does not ease our present turmoil.

One of the most worrisome observed consequences of COVID-19 infection is a blend of cognitive impairment, delirium, and altered mental status. Many of the patients we are treating in the hospital have a relentless case of this COVID brain fog, or what I call zombie mentation, characterized by strange verbalizations or ideations. It is like their brains have been fried a bit. It could be ICU psychosis, an anoxic brain injury consequence of intermittent hypoxia from being on a ventilator for a prolonged period, correspondence to mini strokes, or chemical and hormone derangement. More often, though, it's a new diagnosis, what healthcare workers term *COVID brain*, or *long COVID*. This syndrome involves many symptoms and will require years of studying the long-term effects of COVID-19 infection to understand how to best treat them.

If you are infected and are one of the weak, the predisposed who are layered with comorbidities, you may leave the hospital if you're admitted and live. But in what capacity? Will you have permanent need of supplemental oxygen, caregivers, or a power wheelchair? Will your COVID brain be long term? Will you ever return to your preinfected self? This is the unknown, evermore so giving you a desperate need to prepare yourself for this and other future pathogens by maximizing your health, vitality, and immunity—your pandemic armor.

Although this book was written in the midst of the COVID-19 pandemic, further talk about COVID in particular is not my point. I just wanted to give you a behind-the-scenes glimpse of the happenings inside a hospital during a pandemic. In the end, it doesn't matter what pandemic it is; there have been many pandemics in human history, and there will be many more. It is inevitable.

You do not want to end up being one of the admitted patients during a pandemic—trust me on this one! You do not want to end up dead or one of the undead. You want to be immune, not susceptible. That is why you are reading this book. To learn how to earn pandemic armor and live a life with maximum immunity.

I want to help you don your pandemic armor so you are stronger, healthier, and prepared for the next homicidal pathogen.

To fully grasp the *why* behind the plan, we need to establish the foundational guidelines—the basic ingredients of successful health maintenance and disease prevention.

CHAPTER THREE
THE SUSCEPTIBLE

There is universal commonality among people admitted to a hospital. These common traits, physique trends, disease similarities, and behaviors of typical hospital patients are amplified on the COVID-19 frontline. All these common predispositions are preventable, unhealthy attributes that lead to poor immunity and susceptibility to disease and disability. No matter your race, gender, social class, or creed, if you take preventive action against the most prevalent symptoms, attributes, and behaviors that lead to decreased immunity and hospital admission, then you can maximize your immunity, prevent hospitalization, and ultimately survive a pandemic.

In 2021, the obesity rate of hospital patients is climbing much faster than the global rate. In other words, the global obesity rate is 42 percent and projected to be 50 percent by 2030, but the rate of obesity among the admitted population is much higher. The actual rates are unknown because this predicament is not being researched directly. Based on my calculations of the obesity rate of my patients, I believe the average obesity rate for admitted patients to be at least 60 percent, inching more toward 90 percent on occasion. Being overweight, obese, or morbidly obese is almost always part of a hospital patient's medical history. Why are most hospital patients overweight, obese, morbidly obese, or super-morbidly obese? Because heavy people are entirely comorbid and highly susceptible to sickness, disease, disability, and death. They are the most ruined by the choices they have made throughout their lives.

On occasion I take account of the number of obese patients on my list of therapy patients, and most of the time, 75 percent or higher are obese or morbidly obese. Some days it seems as though the only patients I rehabilitate or observe are overweight or obese and deconditioned. In fact, I almost never, as in maybe once a year, treat a lean, healthy person in the hospital. Those rare cases are typically admitted because of an injury or accident. Hospitals are not for lean, healthy people. Lean, healthy people enter a hospital, are fixed, and are sent home. Fat people linger, progress poorly, and depend on hospitals and doctors to stay alive. Hospitals are for fat, unhealthy, diseased, and disabled people. Most obese people need hospitals to stay alive—at least at some point, usually due to the compounding effects of aging, of growing larger and larger, and of diseases piling up. The hospital is many obese people's second home.

Most hospital workers, including myself, did not go to college to specifically work with and specialize in working with bariatric patients. We want to work in healthcare to help all people in the general sense. The fact is that a healthcare worker has no choice: hospital patients are hospital patients, no matter the body composition. Nowadays, we all have to become experts in handling and caring for bariatric patients because they make up much of the hospital's caseload.

Had we known then what we know now, many healthcare workers might have chosen a different career path—purely because of obesity. This is because obesity is preventable. It is not cancer, dementia, or hemiparesis. Over time, it is human nature for the healthcare worker to lose empathy for people who live with preventable sickness and don't care to treat it themselves. Empathy and sympathy are emotional resources that over time can be drained. Obese patients are extremely difficult to care for, extremely taxing, and a literal heavy burden on the healthcare system. Having an obese patient on a nurse's or therapist's caseload exponentially increases the risk for receiving an on-the-job injury. I do not mean to be callous here. It is simply the truth. I am okay with being the whistleblower on this issue because this issue is going to lead to a mass exodus of healthcare workers to safer career paths like management, door greeting, or non-healthcare small business owner. Obesity must end. People must make healthier decisions and take responsibility for their own self-care, body composition, and physical fitness.

Thousands of traits, behaviors, and comorbidities can harm a hospital patient—or predispose them to admission in the first place—but for the purposes of this book, we are going to focus on the top five. And like the other thousands of preconditions, the top five are all *preventable*.

Could have been treated.

Could have been avoided.

Can be treated now.

Are to some point 100 percent within your control.

The five most prominent traits of a person who is not electively admitted to a hospital are as follows:

10. **Obesity** will destroy your health and lower your immunity, making you susceptible to the consequences of a host of diseases and ailments.
11. **Sarcopenia** is the loss of lean muscle mass, or muscle wasting. Muscle mass is necessary to even have an immune system.
12. **Smoking** has a compounding effect on ill health, disability, and early mortality.

13. **Alcoholism** has the same compounding effect as smoking, minus the respiratory disease but also with mental dysfunction, cognitive impairment, potential disability, and premature demise.

14. **Illicit and prescription drug abuse** is high risk and as death-seeking as a homicidal maniac.

These premorbid conditions host a plethora of other diseases, illnesses, pain, and disability and leave the host susceptible to infection, sickness, and death. If you eliminate just these five traits or behaviors from your life, then you bring your chances of being a hospital patient down to near zero.

The highest predictor of preventable disease, disability, and early death is *obesity*, even more than COVID-19. Obesity is an unnatural yet preventable and treatable state. Earlier, I mentioned the dawn of the Obesiboomers. I created this portmanteau and introduced it in *EXERLEAN* to give light to the worldwide obesity epidemic—or should we say obesity *pandemic*. Obesity is a global phenomenon. The rise of the Obesiboomer generation is only gaining ground.

According to the CDC, over 42 percent of Americans are already obese. Over 18 percent are morbidly obese. Over 83 percent of men and 72 percent of women are overweight or obese. That leaves only 17–28 percent of American adults, depending on gender, who are considered *not* overweight. Sadly, the prevalence of childhood obesity has climbed to over 18.9 percent and continues to rise.

Obesity is defined as having a body mass index, or BMI, over 30. Overweight is having a BMI greater than 25, and morbid obesity is a BMI over 35. A BMI over 40 is astronomically high, severe, and disabling. Seeing patients in the hospital with BMIs in the 50s and 60s is a normal daily occurrence. BMIs this high are termed super-morbid obesity. It is not surprising to see patients with BMIs up to 65 and even higher nowadays. That's two obese people in one, or one morbidly obese person plus another obese person combined. Or three or four healthy people assimilated into one. An abomination of the human body. The human body was never meant to be so fat. Never.

In 1962 the obesity rate was 23 percent. It is predicted that by 2030, 50 percent of Americans will be obese. Obesity is the primary contributing factor in up to four hundred thousand deaths in the US annually. I believe the death rate specifically linked to obesity is much higher considering that obesity is an underlying condition of heart disease, diabetes, strokes, vascular disease, clots, cancers, and infection in general. According to the CDC, the financial burden of obesity on the healthcare system is estimated to be at least $117 billion a year in preventive testing and treatment services—all related to obesity itself. This exceeds the healthcare costs of smoking and alcoholism.

Obesity is the number one contributing factor in obtaining type 2 diabetes, which costs the healthcare system at least $327 billion a year.

Why does obesity matter in consideration of a pandemic?

Because your immunity is destroyed by the plethora of negative health problems and diseases brought about by the preventable state of obesity. What really matters during a pandemic is whether you live or die. How much toilet paper, disinfectant spray, masks, and food you hoard will not help you if you get infected. Only your immune system can save you at that point.

When you get sick, any health problems you are already dealing with—that is, any comorbidities—intensify the disease and suppress the immune system. A comorbidity is a problem with your physical, cognitive, or mental health; your age; a disease; an infection; a deficit;

a disability; or another ailment that suppresses your health. A comorbidity is a condition stacked on another condition, or many other conditions. Comorbidities are the summary of multiple coexisting health problems that become the norm rather than the exception, and that underlie the primary or acute illness, injury, or other emergency at hand. Here's an example: Jim is morbidly obese and contracts the coronavirus. Obesity is a comorbidity underlying Jim's acute illness from the coronavirus infection. Comorbidities plus an acute illness, like in Jim's case, lead to worse outcomes.

Eliminate comorbidities, maximize your pandemic armor.

A little-known health disparity that is rising in the background is sarcopenia. Sarcopenia is the progressive loss of lean muscle mass in relation to aging, sedentary behavior, malnutrition, high biological value protein starvation, lack of bone-on-bone weight bearing, and lack of physical work, all leading to a decaying immune system and the inability to thrive. Sarcopenia is preventable. You could call it the "sitting on your ass watching TV all the time while eating whatever the frick you feel like" disease. Allowing this to remain untreated over time leads to frailty, loss of mobility, loss of self-care, poor quality of life, and looming mortality. Treating it with weight training, cardiovascular exercise, and protein supplementation can maximize your life span and improve your quality of life.

Now the double-edged sword that therapists and nurses have to deal with day in and day out—sarcopenic obesity. A huge person with very little muscle mass underneath all the rolls of fat. A combination of weight and lack of power to move it.

All that excess body fat and not enough muscle to move it: this is the sum of sedentary behavior compounded with obesity and time. Moving an obese patient with low muscle mass is like trying to move a house; it isn't happening, not without a crane. If the obese patient can no longer move themselves, machines are necessary to spare the caregivers from bodily injury. In the hospital we use mini cranes to lift obese patients out of bed and over to a chair or commode. This process takes multiple staff members, leaving other patients waiting longer for their nurses to return to address their needs.

There is a lingering misconception that fat people must have a lot of muscle underneath all that fat because of all that weight they are carrying around. Snakewash! Underneath all that fat is a skinny physique . . . if anything, with less muscle than an active healthy person. The fat person did not get fat because of lifting weights, being active, and eating lean protein and veggies. No! Fat people get fat by consistently eating too much food and living a sedentary lifestyle.

Give credit where credit is due. People who eat lean and light look physically lean and light. People who lift weights have more muscle mass and are stronger. People who engage in daily cardiovascular exercise have heightened activity tolerance, maximum metabolism, and higher cognitive functioning. Vice versa—people who are sedentary have lower endurance, are less tolerant to activity, and are prone to gaining weight. People who do not lift weights or strain their muscles during work or other type of physical resistance will experience atrophy of muscle mass and as a result will be weaker than average. Consuming more food than your metabolic rate, which is lower if you do not exercise or workout, will only lead to weight gain, and that weight gain is not muscle, it is body fat.

Both sarcopenia and obesity are comorbidities that greatly contribute to the susceptibility of sickness, further disease process, decreased life span, and lessened quality of life. In the aging population, both obesity and sarcopenia lead to loss of ability to self-care, as well as progressive loss of functional mobility. Both are preventable. Both can be countered with the necessary treatment. Both lessen your immunity to a pathogen.

The last thing you want to be during a pandemic is dependent on other people for self-care. The mere state of obesity disables typical features of the human body, like the ability to wipe your own butt after a bowel movement. Wiping your own butt is possible because arm length and body proportion are perfectly set up for the hand to reach the wipe zone from almost any approach. Add on a hundred or two pounds of excess body fat, and the glorious feature of wiping is blocked by body mass—obstructed from access. You no wipey, likely need a diapey, or a bidet, and ultimately someone else's hand.

Smoking, alcoholism, and drug abuse are all well-known causes of disease, disability, and early death. There is no need to embellish the facts. They are nonetheless comorbidities that jeopardize your pandemic armor.

Smoking leads to COPD, emphysema, cancer, and susceptibility to respiratory illnesses like pneumonia, chronic bronchitis, and COVID-19. Smoking is the number one cause of lung cancer. Many of the patients we see admitted to the hospital for COVID are smokers or have a history of smoking and are obese. Smoking is obviously preventable and can be instantly eliminated by choice.

Alcohol in small amounts has been shown to be healthy, depending on the type of alcohol, the quantity, and the person. Overusing or overdosing on alcohol leads to liver disease, other organ failure, obesity, brain damage, and some cancers. Alcoholism is an addiction to alcohol that can lead to social, psychological, and physical dysfunction.

During the COVID-19 pandemic, there has been much drinking. Many of us are drinking more alcohol than usual as a coping mechanism to the stress and anxiety that surrounds us. Funny that the stores were unable to keep toilet paper stocked on the shelves, but there has never been a shortage of beer, wine, or liquor.

Drug abuse is on the rise, too. Death from abuse of painkillers is on the rise. Over one hundred people a day die from drug overdoses of various kinds. Cocaine, heroin, methamphetamines, crack, marijuana, opioids, and other illicit drugs are not only highly addictive and unhealthy, but they also decrease one's immunity to viruses, illness, diseases, and death. Drug abuse is 100 percent preventable and treatable if one chooses to do so.

All attributes of unhealth leave a person prone to and burdened with disability, sickness, disease, and likely an earlier-than-normal death. All the unhealthy attributes we have discussed in this chapter are preventable, treatable, and able to be eliminated so you can establish your maximum immunity and pandemic armor. You can be susceptible, or you can be immune. The choice is yours.

CHAPTER FOUR

THE IMMUNE

Who are they?
Where are they?
Why are they?
When are they?
What are they?

The immune are those who seem to never get sick, never need more than preventive healthcare, demonstrate relentless strength and enduring energy, and in general continue to be the highest producers in our society. We all want this for ourselves. We all want to be healthy, productive, immune, strong, and awake. Contributing to the weave that forms our community is a basic human desire—some call it a basic need. Being useful is necessary for self-esteem, personal satisfaction, and vitality. *I am vital.* Who doesn't want to say that?

What is the difference between the immune and the susceptible? The strong and the weak? The lean and the obese? The productive and the unproductive?

The difference is choice. The difference is nothing special that any one of us cannot mimic and live out to harness the power of pandemic armor. The destiny of our desires is at hand, and only the individual has full control over the outcomes simply through the choices they make. The immune choose to be immune, to be in control, and to take action to make it a reality.

To point the responsibility of choice toward anyone or anything other than ourselves is pure irresponsibility—a deflection from self. Deflecting the responsibility of choice is to give the power of control to the external. The external does not give a shit about you and will not work in your best interests. The external world does not have goals that benefit you specifically; you must do the work to achieve your goals for you and you alone. The enemy of choice and control is complaining, blaming, and justifying the situation at hand. To become immune, you must take your power and point it inward, not outward.

Who?

The immune are those who take full responsibility for themselves: their bodies, what they eat and drink, whom they associate with, the choices they make, the actions they take, and the results that follow. My results belong to me and yours are yours; the consequences of personal actions are not shared. The life you realize was born of the seeds you first scattered. I walk in the field I sowed, as do you. You made you what you are today. What you do today, the seeds you plant today, determines who you will be tomorrow.

So that you may become one who is immune, you must enact the same choices of those who are immune. You must adopt their habits, behaviors, and actions, thus becoming immune yourself. The time for transformation is always at hand, so you must choose to change. The metamorphosis from susceptible to immune is up to you. Envision the body you want to walk around in, the energy you want to possess, your heightened sense of self, high self-esteem, the strength to accomplish the miraculous, the power of self-control, and the ability to produce at the highest level.

The immune are athletes, lean eaters, exercisers, workers, and livers of life. They are the innovators, the inventors, the entrepreneurs, the busy bees, the hyperactive, and the contagiously positive and self-believing. The immune person has a will to live as their best possible self. They have relentless enthusiasm for their self-care, their physical composition, their physical abilities, their mental wellness, their cognitive execution, and their level of production. We all have the potential to perform at our best, to eat lean and light, to exercise, to lift weights, to be the hardest worker in the room, and to produce at maximum output. The spark of innovation and ability to achieve our goals is in all of us. The weak suppress this power, while the immune draw from it and act on its influence, intuition, and inclination. If you believe, you can achieve. If you can think it, it is possible. The immune are those who believe they have the power to change their lives however they see fit.

Where?

The immune are at work. They are in the gym. They are working outside. They are taking care of chores. They are moving and grooving to the dance of life. Where they rarely are is on the couch, in a gaming chair, in a recliner, or spacing out. They avoid sedentary and unproductive time. They have work to do, a list of goals to achieve. They are continually unsatisfied with the status quo.

Our heroes are immune. The Olympians, the professional athletes, the superstars, the super rich, the bodybuilders, the fitness icons, the beautiful, the lean, and the happy. They are wherever they need to be to finish their next short-term goal in life, which leads to the next short-term goal, and the next, until the long-term goal is achieved. Then they make new long- and short-term goals and relentlessly follow a step-by-step plan of action. The immune attract their qualities. They build the foundation for and develop their pandemic armor. Where they are is a direct consequence of past decisions, past behavior, and paving their road through life with small incremental goal achievement after goal achievement, finally achieving big wins.

The immune are winners and cannot accept losing unless they know they put forth maximum effort. They will take a loss as a positive learning experience and move forward with the next goal, except now with even more power to win. They do not drag the past with them. They look only to the next thing. They do not accept mediocrity, passivity, or complacency in anything.

And from this point forward, neither will you.

Why?

Why is the immune person the way they are? Why are the susceptible not like them? Because each of their lifestyles usually stems from their parents, the environment that formed them, and the modeling they were forced to adopt without another paradigm to follow.

If your parents are obese, your chances of being obese are almost a guarantee. If your parents smoked during your upbringing, your chances of becoming a smoker are high. The same goes for alcoholism and drug abuse. It is no myth that if you want to know what your husband or wife will look like in the future, look at their parents. If you want to know their hidden qualities or possible future tendencies, look at their parents. Without the willpower to change and the enthusiasm to maintain, it is almost impossible to steer away from our past influences and ego construction. If your parents are bodybuilders or athletic, your chance of living an active life, eating lean, being strong, and knowing discipline is high. If your parents are successful and rich, the same goes for your likelihood of earning wealth and being innovative. If you witnessed entrepreneurship in your youth, it may fuel the flame to become an entrepreneur yourself at some point in your life.

There are those, though, who against all probability, against the external influences of their youth, can change the curve. Regardless of the past, the immune person has inner power. A spark of hope and a relentless drive to change their paradigm if undesired. Many of the richest, most successful, and healthiest people on earth started with a handicap of some sort, forcing them to work harder, which in turn ignited an inner passion to become something extraordinary in spite of their given circumstances.

The immune are immune because they can be, choose to be, and will not settle for less.

When?

Most of the immune are up long before the susceptible. They wake up earliest. They have to take advantage of every possible productive ounce of time. Time is precious to the immune. An hour reclined and watching TV is natural for the susceptible but a sin for the immune. The immune do not have time to waste. They are working, always hyperactive in their chores, and always aware of the value of time.

The immune know not to rest until it is time to sleep. They will sleep the necessary seven to eight hours but not a second more. When it is time to wake up, they wake up. The immune do not snooze; they do not compromise their time or their chance to be productive. They are present in the moment. They are laser-focused on the current action, the next act, and the goal.

The immune are on time. Are reliable and trustworthy. They have earned the respect they receive and the notoriety of their post.

What?

The immune are the best of the best of us. They are the product of their choices, efforts, and accomplishments. They cannot boast binge-watching *The King of Thrones* or the Newflicks TV series. They can, however, reference a plethora of self-help books, successful people, and productive pathways. They can converse about the benefits of weight training and cardiovascular exercise. The immune are the highest producers at work, in the gym, at home, and in the outdoors.

The immune are a prime example of good health. They are the survivors. They are the successors. They have pandemic armor, and you want it too. The focus of this book is to help you transform from wherever you are now to having maximum immunity and pandemic armor. To be prepared for the worst and the best of times. There are going to be many consequences in the process of maximizing your pandemic armor. Like getting in better shape. Improving your health and wellness. Some side effects may include improving your financial potential, increasing your work productivity, earning a better job or position, and increasing your social network.

To help you become one of the immune, we first need to go over some simple action steps. To achieve the atypical outcomes of the immune, you need to learn and enact the foundational qualities of their existence.

Two main sections of this book are devoted to reviewing the building blocks of pandemic armor. The first section, The Foundation for Health, addresses the necessary qualities to maintain basic human life, to at minimum obtain status quo. The basics are a given for the immune; for the susceptible, they are usually neglected. The basics are ingredients for establishing a foundation for building pandemic armor. Building your pandemic armor on a faulty foundation will only lead to catastrophic failure. The second section, Maximum Immunity, is a guide to maximizing your immunity and earning pandemic armor.

By truly nurturing and caring for yourself, you can build a fortress upon this rock of solidarity.

THE FOUNDATION FOR MAXIMUM HEALTH

CHAPTER FIVE

PARENTAL ADVICE

A *portal of entry* or *exodus* is the weak spot in your armor. It's usually a hole, literally, in your skin—a doorway to the inside of your body. The most common portals that a pathogen will enter are through the mouth, nose, eyes, anus, vagina, urethra, nail beds, ears, or defects in the protective skin layer—wounds. Through these portals, the pathogen can enter, infect the host, manifest itself— replicate—and ultimately leave to find another host through contact (touch), droplet (spit), or air (breath). This is the disease transmission pathway.

At some point in our childhood, we are taught basic life skills and self-care by parents, teachers, and other mentors to prevent a pathogen from entering one of our portals. *Brush your teeth! Wash your hands! Take a shower! Clean your room!* These foundational qualities of being an independent human being are learned in childhood, developed in youth, and mastered in the teenage years. The basics allow us to move forward in our adult lives to bigger and better territory without an afterthought. The immune do not give thought to self-care; they just do it. These subconscious jobs are done without failure or regret; they are eternal unless taken away by poor health, poor decision-making, or disability. The ability to self-care is so second nature that most people take it for granted, and consequently, it is the most missed of all physical abilities when lost to disability.

The richest man in the world, crippled by disease, would pay everything to restore his ability to walk, to dress, to wash his feet. He regrets not doing more when he could have to build his health rather than pave the pathway for disease and disability.

Her majesty Queen of Bora Bora, stricken with disabling obesity, has lost her mobility and the ability to self-care—she constantly prays to trade all the royalty and riches for the lightweight, lean, and able body she once had. She lives in regret. Hers is a life spent deflecting her pain and anguish to external sources rather than taking control of the wheel and righting the wrong.

You cannot wish for, hope for, or conjure a spell to remove the preventable features that will inevitably slow you down, disable you, and eventually kill you. God will not melt off your fat for you. Fat does not get burned magically or without action on your part. The power to melt off body fat is already yours. It is your God-given metabolism and your muscles that can burn calories at rest and even more when you engage them in manual labor, work, or exercise. Your metabolism is your birthright, your power, and you can use it to melt away your debilitating body fat.

Nobody can make you quit smoking. Only you have this power. When you smoke, you choose to smoke. When you quit smoking, you choose to quit. The cigarette or magazine ad does not put the cigarette in your mouth and light it up—you pull the trigger, you flick the Bic. The drug dealer did not make you taste the drug—you made the decision to pop the pill, smoke the crank, or inject the poison. Nobody can make you quit taking drugs. This power lies in you. The stress, your ex, or your boss did not make you drink too much alcohol. You hold the cup, bring it to your mouth, taste what's in it, swallow it, and put it into your body. Unless you are a helpless baby, you are not fed, you self-feed. What you can do is take the first step and then the next. Remove the behaviors, traits, and physical attributes that create unhealthy habits and cause addiction, sickness, disability, and eventually death. You have all the power to change everything you think, feel, and do. When you do this hinges on you. Where you do it does not matter. Do it whenever and wherever you are right now.

Self-Care

When I started working as an occupational therapist, *self-care* was the primary focus area in the practice of occupational therapy, but the term was little known to the rest of the world. OTs were and are sometimes still belittled for this. "Self-care, that's stupid," people would reply when we brought it up. Well, nowadays every self-help guru, wellness coach, and nutritionist has grabbed on to this OT focus area and is maximizing its use for their benefit, taking the focus away from the real meaning behind the term. Self-care in the original sense is not going to a spa, getting a massage, or going on a hike. Mindfulness, relaxation, and green drinks are not self-care; they are health tools that help you maximize self-care potential.

Self-care. It's the stuff like washing behind the ears, brushing your teeth, and wiping your butt.

Come on, John! What the hell—self-care! Don't waste my time, you might be thinking. Trust me. Whether or not you think you know what self-care is, whether you think you self-care sufficiently, or whether you think this topic is unimportant, stay focused. Unless you are already wearing the armor of maximum immunity, unless you are well prepared for the next zombie apocalypse—learn and prepare. You suffer from susceptibility because you didn't listen to your parents, disrespected authority, or in some other capacity failed to adopt the basics of self-care when you should have. There are missing ingredients in your foundational upbringing that are preventing you from completing the recipe for developing immunity. It is possible that you had an atypical upbringing and that situations beyond your control left you lacking the integral life skills—or ingredients—for formulating pandemic armor. I know this because I was dealt this hand and I paid for it—thank God I paid for it. For if I did not, I would not have my pandemic armor today.

Moments of opportunity come to us throughout our lives. The basics of self-care come in our youth and cease to be taught thereafter. If you miss the boat, you have to swim like hell to catch back up to everyone else making the journey to the lands of promise and success. You cannot be successful if you cannot self-care; it is the bare-bones expectation of our civilization. You cannot have maximum immunity if you cannot even take care of yourself.

Some of us fail to harness the power of self-care, possibly because we don't fully comprehend it. To repair this inequality in self-care, people like me—occupational therapists and personal trainers, as well as doctors—have the expertise, knowledge, and skill to help you fill the gaps in your foundation with good cement.

Let's rebuild your foundation and make it solid as a rock. From your foundation, we will build your pandemic armor.

As an occupational therapist working in the acute care hospital setting, I have seen everything under the sun. Healthcare workers in direct patient care see shit that would turn your stomach inside out. These encounters happen on most days. Had the cloak of benevolence not been masking the raw truth of direct patient care, many of us would have steered clear of a healthcare occupation. In healthcare schools, the reality of picking at wounds, wiping other people's butts, lifting fat people, or treating happenstance scabies is not fully realized until it is too late and you're locked into a high-paying career that was expensive to obtain.

Self-care encompasses the private to the blatant and sometimes public actions of taking care of our body. We complete some of our self-care in public, like washing our hands and face, brushing our hair, brushing our teeth, putting on makeup, or in some cases toileting—for guys using urinals side by side or anyone using a toilet stall. In all these displays of public self-care, we can either see, hear, or smell others in the act. The private and personal self-care we usually deal with at home or behind closed doors includes bathing, getting dressed, toileting ourselves, putting on deodorant, and cleaning our nostrils, eyes, belly button, butt crack, and nails.

In the hospital, we see the susceptible majority, many with a resumé of poor self-care. If you want to be sick, become a frequent flyer to a hospital, hobble throughout your day, and lust for better physical ability, poor self-care will get you there at some point.

What is poor self-care? Let's go over some examples.

For one, the inability to wipe your butt, or self-wiping with poor quality. We call this job the act of *toileting* in healthcare, and it is a big issue. I'd say more than 75 percent of patients cannot wipe their butts after a bowel movement. The nurse wipes your butt for you. This is the lowest of the low. The bottom-of-the-barrel duties. Throughout the day, first thing in the morning, after a break, before and after lunch, and just before going home, someone wipes a patient's butt for them. This is the shit that makes healthcare workers think twice about the career they have chosen. To consider something—anything—that does not involve wiping someone else's normally suffocated, now-exposed, obese, malodorous, hairy, and disgusting butt crack. There are no healthy butt cracks admitted to a hospital. Most people working outside a healthcare setting have no idea how good they have it. If you complain about your current job, try doing the work of a nurse for a day. Wipe someone else's ass! Clean it up real good. Your feelings about your job will improve tenfold.

Another important self-care job is bathing. In the hospital setting, we see a crazy number of patients who have not bathed in months, and before that, it was just as infrequent. We see patients who have lichens growing on their skin that cannot be picked off; it is part of their skin. The armpits, the inner thighs, between the toes, the belly button, the peroneal area, in between folds of fat, under breasts, behind the ears, the double chin area, and your private parts are confined in the depths of your underwear, which are underpants for many, and that which lies in the darkness cannot breathe.

Sounds like a line in a horror movie.

These areas build up sweat, excrement, dead skin cells, and toxins rather quickly.

Dead cells, toxins, excrement . . . am I describing a zombie here?

These areas of the body need to be cleaned in warm, soapy water daily. The susceptible do not bathe as often as they should, though, leaving them prone to poor hygiene, skin discoloration, brown clumping due to compounding layers of dead skin cells, offensive body odor, greasy and stinky hair, itching, acne breakouts, puss, groin rashes, painful intertrigo (yeast infection and skin inflammation), skin funguses, scum between the toes, and other diseases and infections.

Oral care is another important area of self-care that if neglected can do much more damage than the predicament of bad breath or cavities.

Did you know that poor oral hygiene can lead to dental infections that will kill you, as well as sinus infections? Your oral cavity and sinus passages are less than an inch away from the blood-brain barrier, which is semipermeable. Left untreated, bacteria from a toxic sinus or oral infection can cross the blood-brain barrier and kill you. Poor oral care has also been found to increase the risk of dementia and Alzheimer's disease, and it can amplify other comorbidities like heart disease, cancer, and diabetes.

Do you have mouth pain, bleeding, swelling, discoloration, tongue abnormalities, growths, or receding gum lines? These are all symptoms of poor oral self-care.

Getting dressed is basic self-care. Humans are not meant to be naked on the earth. We do not have thick fur to protect us from the ultraviolet rays of the sun, the subzero temperatures of winter, and the other harsh elements of mother nature, like hurricanes, tornadoes, drought, earthquakes, and volcanic eruptions. If we did not have clothing to add external protection, the sharp claws and teeth of meat-eating animals would have no difficulty tearing into us and taking us down. Clothing protects us from getting scratches, scrapes, puncture wounds, and other injuries, which can lead to an opening in the skin, a portal of entry for infection. Clothing also protects our skin from environmental toxins like poison ivy, poison oak, and stinging nettles.

Lesson One: "Wipe Your Own!"

Can you wipe your butt? If you can, is it difficult to do? More importantly, if it is wiped, is it clean and hygienic? Guess what? Many people cannot wipe their own butt, leading to poor health consequences.

The peroneal area is the area that encompasses our crotch, groin, and everything in between to the top of our butt crack. Left unattended frequently, this area is susceptible to poor hygiene, which in turn leaves you prone to the results of poor hygiene—urinary tract and other infections like *E. coli*, enterococcus, *C. diff*, and diarrheal parasites, and aside from potential infections you can end up with open wounds, anal discomfort, itching, disease, and bacterial residue that can spread illness through contact to other people.

Did you know that most diarrheal illnesses attributed to buffets or other communal food environments are due to eating shit residue from someone's poorly washed or unwashed post-bowel-movement-wiping hands that grabbed the potato salad serving spoon just before you did?

No shit! Many diarrheal illnesses are caused by eating shit—literally—and it is not your shit.

Washing your hands before you eat gets rid of possible shit that you are about to put in your mouth when you eat, pick your teeth, or bite your nails.

Like other areas, the peroneal area should be washed in warm, soapy water daily. Parents teach their children to take a daily shower for this basic reason. During the day you may have gas, may shart (a little shit expelled during a fart), or have a bowel movement (a BM). If you don't wipe it, you leave it there. If you don't wash your hands thoroughly, then it may remain on your hands. When you go to eat, it attaches to your finger foods. Do not eat shit.

Poop is a waste product evacuated from the human body; it is composed of stuff our body does not want. According to the United Nations Department of Economic and Social Affairs, one gram of poop contains ten million viruses, one million forms of bacteria, one thousand parasitic cysts, and one hundred worm eggs. One gram! That's like two raisins. Shit needs to be removed from the body. According to Aaron Glatt, chair of medicine at South Nassau Communities Hospital and spokesperson for the Infections Disease Society of America, "In terms of hygiene, it is unacceptable" not to wipe. "Find something to clean yourself off with. . . . Use water or leaves. Do everything possible." Take this gem of advice and make sure that the leaves are not poison ivy. Like I learned at Boy Scout camp: "Leaves of three, let it be."

The consistency of poop can worsen the situation, especially for women who are more prone than men to get urinary or vaginal infections. A poopy anus is very close to the vagina and the urethra, which are portals of entry for infection. "If you have loose stool, it can spread further," says Philip M. Tierno, a NYU School of Medicine professor. Loose stooling or diarrhea can seep into clothing and break through to the outside environment more easily. Now your feces is on the chair you sat on. The next person gets your shit on their pants and possibly unknowingly on their hands, and then they forget to wash their hands before eating popcorn. Now your poop is possibly making another person sick.

Norovirus, otherwise known as gastroenteritis, is a highly contagious pathogen spread typically through communal food opportunities like cafeterias, buffets, and nursing homes. Usually, norovirus is derived from someone else's shit getting in your stomach and making you sick. Maybe it got on a food handle from someone else's poopy hands, or maybe the food preparation laborer washed their hands poorly after taking a dump—then you touched the handle and didn't wash your hands before eating. *C-difficile* (*C. diff* for short) is another highly infectious bacterium that spreads through poop spores in the environment, on surfaces, or on objects when people who are infected do not wash or poorly wash their hands, contaminating anything they touch, including through food handling.

Wipe it off with toilet paper, baby wipes, or a washcloth. If you have a bidet, use it. When your peroneal area is clean and hygienic, wash your hands until no more specks of bowel remain. Whatever you do, do not allow shit to remain in any capacity on your skin—ever. And for the love of all things "sane-itary," do not eat it.

Lesson Two: Wash Your Hands.

Handwashing frequently throughout the day is one of the easiest and best actions you can do to protect yourself and others from getting sick. Per the Centers for Disease Control and Prevention (CDC), there are key times to wash your hands:

- Before, during, and after preparing food.
- Before and after eating.
- Before and after caring for a sick person who is vomiting or has diarrhea.
- Before and after treating a cut or wound.
- After using the toilet.
- After changing dirty diapers or cleaning a child who has gone to the bathroom.
- After blowing your nose, coughing, or sneezing.
- After touching an animal, animal feed, or animal waste.
- After handling pet food or pet treats.
- After touching garbage.

The general rule of thumb for good handwashing is to use warm water and scrub with soap for at least twenty seconds. Another way to disinfect your hands if a sink is unavailable is to use at least 60 percent alcohol-based hand sanitizer.

Lesson Three: Take a Shower or Bath Daily.

Some parts of your body may not need *daily* bathing, but other parts do, like underneath your breasts, your armpits, in between skin folds, your groin, your butt crack, your peroneal area, and your feet. You do not want to have an offensive body odor, greasy hair, or a dirty appearance.

Lesson Four: Brush and Floss Twice Daily.

Brush and floss your teeth at least twice a day with a soft-bristled brush per the American Dental Association (ADA). We already discussed the possible negative health consequences of poor oral hygiene, including death.

Lesson Five: Maintain Your Grooming and General Hygiene Self-Care.

Grooming and general hygiene include things like getting a haircut when necessary, keeping fingernails and toenails trimmed and clean, maintaining skin health on the bottoms of feet and palms of hands, cleaning your belly button, cleaning the corners of your eyes, cleaning your ears, and monitoring your skin for defects or possible portals of entry.

Lesson Six: Wear Clean Clothing Daily.

"Change your clothes." That was our parents' gripe—and for good reason. Wearing dirty clothes is a precursor for illness. Clothing that is not cleaned regularly starts to build up germs and bacteria that can cause the wearer to get yeast infections, urinary tract infections, jock itch or other genital fungi, athlete's foot, bad acne, stinky body odor, and other sicknesses.

Did you know that the average human sheds thirty thousand to forty thousand dead skin cells a day? That is roughly one to two pounds of dead skin cells a year. Add sweat to all that dead skin; the average person sweats up to ten to fourteen liters per day. Sweat is made up of 99 percent water and 1 percent salt, fat, ammonia, and urea. Men do not sweat more than women; this is a myth. The amount of sweat and dead-skin-cell buildup has *nothing* to do with gender but everything to do with body size. The bigger you are, the more you shed and sweat. The bigger the woman than the man—the more the woman sweats than the man. The bigger the man than the woman—the more the man sweats than the woman.

Wear clean clothes! Disinfect your shoes!

IADLs

After basic self-care, our parents teach us higher-level activities of daily living. In healthcare, we call these jobs instrumental activities of daily living (IADLs). IADLs include basic living jobs like making your bed, cleaning your room, food prep, housecleaning, laundry, and taking out the garbage.

Living in a clean environment is necessary for healthy living. Did you know that living in a dirty, cluttered home increases all residents' levels of anxiety and stress and can lead to poor concentration? It can also make you feel overwhelmed and out of control. A dirty home can damage both your physical and mental health. Research has shown that hoarders end up living in isolation and have a higher tendency of over-eating and becoming obese. Do not hoard.

Dust buildup can cause allergies due to dust mites and pet dander. Homes that have animal excrement in them can lead to human contamination and illnesses. Dog, cat, mouse, or other animal feces contain parasites, pestilence, and disease. Just smelling animal feces is associated with diarrhea, hantavirus, trachoma, digestive dysfunction, growth faltering, infections, and other health conditions.

A dirty bed can host dead skin, sweat, urine, feces, other body fluids, and dust mites, and if you let your pet sleep in your bed, then add in animal mites, ringworm, and anything else attached to their feet or fur, like feces, urine, and other outside elements. A dirty bed also makes you susceptible to bedbugs and scabies. Please, wash your pillowcases, comforter, and pillows regularly, at least once a week.

The car is another place we spend time in that can make us sick. Is your car old? Does it sit outside? Did you know that mice love to make nests in cars? And with that, leave feces in your engine compartment, heater and AC venting, interior floor, and hatchback or trunk space? Do you vacuum out your car and keep it clean at all times?

I have seen two patients admitted to the hospital after getting infected with hantavirus, which was acquired while cleaning out their filthy cars ridden with mouse poop.

Mold is another danger for humans. Moldy surfaces release spores into the environment when breathed into your lungs, which can make you sick. Research by the University of Nottingham showed that more than half of cars have unhealthy and potentially fatal pathogens like *E. coli* and MRSA (methicillin-resistant Staphylococcus aureus). Staphylococcus can cause food poisoning and necrotizing pneumonia. Please, keep your vehicle spick-and-span, sanitized, and mold- and rodent-free.

Now imagine an average thin person who does not properly bathe, wears the same dirty clothes day after day, does not change their bedding regularly, drives in a filthy car, and brushes their teeth once a week. They might smell bad, have greasy hair, get sick from the dust in the car, and become ill if they have a wound that allows a pathogen to enter their skin—but the probability of infection is low. Okay, now add one comorbidity to this person, obesity. This situation just became a whole lot worse. Now this person has folds of skin that are building up dead skin and fungus, and it's likely they are having more difficulty wiping their butt. Now add another comorbidity to this obese dirty person, smoking. Now this person has compromised respiratory function and is much more susceptible to getting sick from dust, mold, and other airborne pathogens. Now add alcoholism, which leads to the slow death of their internal organs, including their brain. They now have multiple comorbidities that make them very susceptible to getting an illness or disease, and a higher chance of becoming disabled or dying sooner than later. This person has a poor foundation for surviving an illness, let alone a *novel* coronavirus pandemic.

Novel means that the pathogen has never been experienced or identified in humans and therefore has no known treatment protocol or medicine to reduce symptoms. COVID-19 is thinning the herd, and most who are killed by it have multiple comorbidities. That is how it became a global pandemic. COVID-19 is a novel coronavirus and extremely contagious. We have many obese and sedentary people, smokers, alcoholics, and susceptible elderly people on this earth, and they are the majority of those dying from COVID-19.

It is not difficult to acknowledge comorbidities in ourselves. Comorbidities are obvious to oneself as well as external observers. Obesity is a clear and present danger. Sarcopenia is obvious weakness, frailty, and susceptibility. Smoking, drinking, and doing drugs are well-known risks and statistically harmful. Why does a person persist in lacking self-care, overeating unhealthy foods, being sedentary, smoking cigarettes, consuming too much alcohol, and doing illicit drugs? Why is it that most of us resist change to get better? Why do so many of us try to lose weight and fail? Why do our efforts to finish New Year's resolutions peter out? Why do we quit our diets? Why do we quit exercising and working out? Why is it so hard to win in the mission of improving ourselves?

Why is it so easy, almost subconscious, to continue engaging in the harmful, unhealthy, and rote activities that we know are so? Why is it so easy to take the path of least resistance, to procrastinate with the work, to forgo the effort, to quit? Why is it so easy that we don't even have to try to do the things we want so badly to quit doing? Most of the mindless self-harm happens at exactly that—the place of mindlessness, your subconscious or unconscious mind.

What is it that stops our efforts toward positive health transformation?

It is our mind—the CEO of our company.

CHAPTER SIX
THE CEO

Your mind sets the stage for your life as it has unfolded today and will unfold tomorrow. Your past actions laid the foundation on which you construct your life today. Your thoughts are your presence at this very moment; they come from your brain, your soul, and they are your connection to the body, and from the body all external elements—other brains, other souls, all things living and dead in the universe. Your health status today is the result of thoughts that have manifested to behaviors, which direct decision-making and actions predetermined by your CEO. Yesterday created the results you live today. There is only this moment. At this time, what you choose to focus on, to think about, to act on is all that counts. Presently you enact your life, feel your feelings, do it, need it, want it, take action to obtain, achieve, or earn it—or you don't. Yesterday is over, unchangeable, regrettable. There is hope for tomorrow. Your future depends on everything you do, think, and say now—because today is all that matters.

Did you know that all things living and inanimate have a vibration, that they give off and accept a signal, connecting to all other things in the universe? Aristotle called this connection the *aether*, and in physics it's referred to as the hypothetical *luminiferous ether*. *Merriam-Webster* defines the ether as "the sky—used especially when describing electronic signals that travel through the air." In the world-famous book *Think and Grow Rich*, author Napoleon Hill states, "He should have told us that the ether in which this little earth floats, in which we move and have our being, is a form of energy moving at an inconceivably high rate of vibration, and that the ether is filled with a form of universal power which ADAPTS itself to the nature of the thoughts we hold in our minds; and INFLUENCES us, in natural ways, to transmute our thoughts into their physical equivalent."

Napoleon Hill describes our connection to the universe as being of vibration, which is energy. Through this energy or vibration, we can manifest thoughts into external reality. If you think it and believe you can achieve it, then what was once thought will become a product or a result that unfolds into your life. Some refer to this as belief in self, or the seeds you sow. Or maybe it is purely self-control with added discipline and execution. The word *think* in the title of his book describes the premise of all reality. If you did not think, you would be mindless, the living dead. *Think* of being rich, and you will *grow rich*. This concept seems unrealistic at first, but it is the basis of all teachings that come from our mentors, gurus, teachers, and usually the most famous, most successful people in history. I have not met or read about a famous Olympian, martial artist, actor, author, entrepreneur, business tycoon, inventor, innovator, bodybuilder, or another form of winner who does not describe the continuous use of visualization, belief in self, relentless enthusiasm, fearless focus, and positive affirmations in their path to victory. They believe they have already won, so they do just that—win.

Through thoughts, they send the vibrations to their bodies and the universe of execution, winning, and finally victory. From thought to memory, they program their mind and its connection to the body, mapping future movements and visualizing all execution before delivery of the goods and services. As an example: the punch would be the product of the *service* of boxing. The *goods* can be the invention of the next computer chip or the next recipe for fried chicken wings, and the *service* would be the process of delivering, or selling, the goods. The goods and services can unfold as almost anything a human can produce, from designing a new management model to breaking the world record for physical performance in the Olympics, winning the next UFC fight, taking first place and the overall in a bodybuilding competition, or executing some other feat of superhuman power or innovation.

Like radio waves, cellular signals, or satellite signals, there is a medium for everything to connect. Maybe it is vibration, maybe it has another name and exists at the subatomic level. Atoms are broken down into protons, neutrons, and electrons. We cannot see these things, but they are scientifically proven to exist. They were just theories until we were able to make the microscope powerful enough to visualize them. The same may be for the ether.

Take food, for instance. Food gives us an intense multisensory experience through visualization—colors, flavor and taste, temperature, touch, chemical reactions, sound, and transfer of energy through proteins, sugars, and fats. Food gives off vibrations of varying intensities. One such food is the Szechuan pepper. In a study done by the National Institutes of Health (NIH), the Szechuan pepper gives off a somatosensory effect, boosting taste likely through the medium of touch. Since this is so, the theory of vibrations connecting all things might not be so unpalatable.

The God particle was a theory until in 2012 scientists confirmed its existence. The God particle was discovered by English physicist Peter Higgs and others in 1964. According to Higgs, the God particle is an invisible universal field that gave mass to all matter right after the Big

Bang. Maybe there is something smaller than the God particle we have yet to discover, something that would explain the ether. This idea would not go against the perpetual unfolding of discoveries over time.

The ether is a theory, sort of like the soul—there's no scientific proof for a soul, but we know it exists because there is a connection. Call it faith, karma, or intuition, it is the tie that binds at the smallest yet undiscovered level. The first human action from the soul is thought. This is why your thoughts are the seeds for the product of your life. Your thoughts control your actions, your behaviors, and your health.

Have you ever called out to the universe, to God, to nothing—and received an answer? Through an amazing series of events, your wish, your longing, your prayer, your ask is presented to you miraculously. This may not be a coincidence. Many believe that such occurrences are the direct result of the ask-and-answer paradigm, which I have experienced many times over the course of my life. Answers are delivered in an inexplicable, supernatural manner. This may be the direct product of what was once a thought or projection from the mind. On a level that is scientifically unexplainable as of yet, our mind connects you and me to all things. Our thoughts have substance—energy, which in turn fosters a communication path to everything in the universe. This form of interconnectedness takes place at an invisible level, to the people around us, and all other things connected through them. Whether you call it the law of attraction, the luminiferous ether, or vibrations, it is connected to us through the power of thought.

Your thoughts—your mind—are the CEO of your physical body, all its organs, blood, hormones, chemical reactions, and other physiological phenomena that give you life. If the CEO has the wrong thoughts and orders the wrong decisions, the company will fail. Your body is its own unique corporation from the brain, through the circulation of blood and transmission of nerve impulses through your organs right down to the skin on the soles of your feet. The CEO is the *guiding light* of the corporation. The precursor to the economy within.

The power of light is described in lumens. A lumen is a unit of measurement for the brightness of light, otherwise referred to as candle power, or radiance. This is the same radiance described in the word *luminiferous*, as in the luminiferous ether. Your thoughts are your body's *guiding light*. Your thoughts can make you get sick just as your thoughts can make you get better. This is the power of thought. It creates long-lasting effects because everything you do leans toward the thought. Negative thoughts and actions attract negative results. Positive thoughts and actions, therefore, deliver positive results.

As the CEO of your body, you command all things your body does. Only you have this power. No other person controls you or your mind. Your thoughts are the first level of your health because they determine the strength of your pandemic armor. Just as a seed grows into a tree, your thoughts are seeds that grow into your life as it is today. Your health hinges on you executing health-conscious thoughts and positive actions toward your wellbeing.

Your physical body is the product of past thoughts, behaviors, actions, and results compounded over time. If you are unhealthy, it is your doing. If your immunity is low, this is your doing too. You are the CEO, and all thoughts you command, including those that lead to behaviors and subsequent actions of overeating, eating unhealthy foods, and being sedentary, are your responsibility. Obesity is the product of past thoughts and actions. If you engage in unhealthy actions like drinking too much alcohol, smoking cigarettes, doing drugs, living sedentary, or socializing with losers who do not support your wellbeing, then you are the living product of those decisions.

Just like a failing corporation needs to replace a bad CEO with a good one to return the corporation to greatness, you too need to get rid of your bad CEO—your bad thoughts. These bad thoughts become habits, eventually leaving you susceptible to illness.

Although you cannot fire yourself from the CEO position, you can transform your CEO mindset and actions. You have the power of free will, and with this power, the ability to change yourself at any time you so choose.

Unless you are on your deathbed, it is never too late to change. To say otherwise is to engage in the poison of life—complaining, blaming, making excuses, and justifying your perpetually staying the same. Being susceptible to illness and disease is a symptom. Susceptibility is an unhealthy symptom. A symptom that change is necessary—that transformation is paramount to survival. This is a time for transformation. Forming good self-care routines, adopting lean eating habits, and behaving in a positive, healthy manner all start with a thought. A thought is a seed that when planted expands into something—grows stronger, matures, and produces more thoughts. It is time to plant the seeds of positive change. Time to behave in a way conducive to adopting healthy living routines. Time to self-care at a premium level.

Your body and its immune system are the product of your actions that originate in thought. To believe you can transform from a susceptible person to an immune survivor, you must think it, then act accordingly to make it so.

What you think is triggered by your surroundings, the last person you talked to, the next person on the list, pain, discomfort, pleasure, desire, and you. Any one of us has the power to instantly change a thought pattern into another. If emotion is involved, however, which is usually the case, it is more difficult to change. Emotion is a feeling. You have control of both emotions and thoughts, but less so of emotions.

Emotions are the result of psychological and physical reactions that can influence our thoughts and behaviors. Emotions are the precursors to our personality, dictate our mood, and provide the basic motivation to engage in life. They have a powerful influence on our thoughts. In their study "How emotions inform judgment and regulate thought," NIH researchers acknowledge this influence by concluding that "affect and emotion are pervasive influences on human judgment and thought."

To be able to control your thoughts, you must be able to regulate your emotions as well. Yes, you can choose how you feel and how you react to how you are feeling. As you will it, so will it be. Free will is your God-given gift. From this right, you claim ownership in all your decisions, feelings, and thoughts.

Many people who are obese, smoke, do drugs, and drink too much are susceptible because they live a life led by emotions. A 2010 study found that emotional issues such as depression, anxiety, and sadness are often associated with obesity. The study found that obese people were 55 percent more likely to develop depression compared to non-obese people. Depression and anxiety are both associated with being sedentary, eating too much, eating unhealthy fat-laden and sugary foods, and over time becoming obese. So, my question is: Did obesity lead to depression, or did emotional instability or negative emotions in general lead to behaviors that cause obesity? Likely both cases are true. A person who is emotionally weak or whose emotions predispose them to overeating and sedentary behavior will eventually become obese, and an obese person can develop depression much easier than a lean person purely due to obesity's unwanted, unhealthy, and negative connotations.

Anxiety and stress are the typical justifications for smoking cigarettes and drinking alcohol. Self-medicating, some call it, to relieve unwanted feelings and moods. Tobacco, drugs, and alcohol incapacitate our thinking, usually leading to poor judgment and reckless behavior that raises the risk of crime, violence, self-harm, and other regrettable acts.

There are healthy ways to deal with anxiety, stress, pain, and suffering, like weight training; cardiovascular exercise; eating light and lean; placing oneself in an environment of happiness; patience, and positive reinforcement; associating with motivated, successful, happy, and healthy people; reading self-help books; going on vacations; meditating; and finding solace outdoors. These can be great tools for finding one's center. All these self-care options and more are at your fingertips, and none will lead to reckless thoughts, poor judgment, or regret.

By identifying the feelings or emotions of anxiety and stress, which generate from the *subconscious* or *unconscious*, we can regulate and manage them by *consciously* choosing positive reinforcing thoughts, which will counter the path that negative emotions drive us toward. The ability to consciously identify thoughts that are derived from emotion takes maturity and skill, which usually comes with age and wisdom. When negative thoughts are identified, they must be replaced with positive reinforcing thoughts. This takes practice, and it becomes easier as you develop this skill set.

Anger is a dangerous emotion that can lead to rage, violence, crime, and imprisonment. It is often associated with blaming and is the feeling or emotion that develops from someone else's unwanted actions. Anger is a negative emotional state that is perceived as hostile and nonproductive; it's an enemy to other people, work environments, or social gatherings.

Anger can also be channeled as a physical and emotional response for coping with stress, anxiety, and fear. Angry outbursts, yelling, or hitting some*thing* can release tension and calm your nerves. To ensure this emotion is not counterproductive to positive transformation, you can easily treat it with constructive modalities such as weight training, cardiovascular exercise, punching a heavy bag, and consciously replacing anger-derived negative thoughts with positive calming thoughts. This free will is a skill set you can develop with purpose, practice, and discipline.

Aside from treating negative emotions constructively, you must train yourself to replace negative emotions with positive ones. Positive emotions that will help you succeed in life include happiness, confidence, love, patience, enthusiasm, excitement, gratitude, and grace. "I can do this," "Have no fear," "I will succeed," "I choose to do it," and "I am happy" are just some examples of positive reinforcing thoughts you can choose to feel. Overeating or eating unhealthy comfort foods, on the other hand, are usually based on subconscious thoughts and lead us astray.

I mentioned *modalities* as a way to help redirect your anger. Modalities are tools that treat symptoms like pain, discomfort, and weakness, or emotions like anger, tension, anxiety, sadness, and stress. For example, massage therapy is a modality for treating tension, easing muscle cramps, and relieving stress. Weight training can extinguish anger, rage, and stress. Aerobic exercise can enhance an enlightened state of emotion and treat sadness or depression. If it can help heal your pain, relinquish your emotional turmoil, and turn a negative state into a positive one, let's treat it as a modality. You can be your modality. Your emotions, thoughts, and actions are modalities if they lead you to positive healing and maximal immunity.

Every emotion and every thought you experience is transmitted from thought to thought, through the ether, through vibrations interacting with other vibrations, or through some other frequency. Your thoughts and feelings influence the universe and have a direct impact on the products of your life. If you think you will lose, you will. If you are stressed, you will attract stress. If you are depressed, you will attract depression, and if you are angry, you will attract anger. You will be unsuccessful in life if you are led by negative thoughts and emotions, if you self-medicate with alcohol or drugs to deal with stress, and if you operate on a subconscious level of thought and action. Your pandemic armor will be susceptible if you are an angry, stressed, anxious, or depressed person. Negative thoughts and emotions leave you susceptible to illness, disease, obesity, addiction, and disability.

On the contrary, positive emotions and conscious positive thinking lead to good health, wellness, social cohesion, friendship, attraction, boosted work productivity, and maximal success. A successful transformation comes on a positive level, not a negative level. An unsuccessful transformation is led by negative thoughts and emotions; it is typical of those who follow the path of failure, the path to addiction, or the path to early disease and mortality. Your connection to the universe hinges on your emotions, and from that, your thoughts. Do you want think and grow fatter, think and do drugs, think and drink alcohol, think and be sedentary? Or do you want to think and grow stronger, think and grow healthier, think and grow wiser, think and win, think and be successful—think and build up your pandemic armor?

From the thoughts and emotions of your CEO come your behaviors. Behavior is how you display yourself to the world. It can be of action or inaction, audible or silent. It can operate subconsciously or consciously. Because behavior stems from emotion and thought, it is also controllable by your right of free will.

Children learn how to behave through classical conditioning, modeling, positive reinforcement, negative reinforcement, punishment, reward, trial, and error. Through these methods, parents are responsible for ensuring their children behave in socially acceptable ways. Appropriate behavior is a basic necessity for a child to be successful in school, in relationships, and in their future adult lives. To the detriment of many kids, some parents are incompetent at the job of parenting. As a result, their children fail to learn the necessary skills of behavior regulation and are therefore susceptible to negative returns from their environment.

The skills for emotional regulation and behavior modification can be learned later in life through teachers, mentors, trial-and-error self-experience, and fast-tracked through studying self-help books like this one, taking courses to learn new skills, or seeking expert mentorship. It is never too late to learn new life skills. Don't fret if your parents fucked you up. If you had no parents. If you're in a state of confusion, failure, expulsion, or destitution because of the way your parents or the system molded you. If you fail socially, in relationships, and in interpersonal communication because your mentors were shit. You must self-teach, self-care, and self-seek the type of person you want to become. Change is doable. If you want it, you can achieve it, so long as you are willing to change. Your vision of future you is on the horizon. Let's start with the way you behave.

According to *Merriam-Webster*, behavior is "the way in which someone conducts oneself or behaves; anything that an organism does involving action and response to stimulation; the response of an individual, group, or species to its environment; the way in which something functions or operates." Behavior is the most important element of one's self-control, social conduct, personal interactions, and productivity. Outward behavior is a response that originates from underlying emotions and thoughts. When a person behaves the same way to a certain stimulus for long enough, that response becomes routine.

Through routines, we subconsciously develop habits of behavior, which leads to a flow state of performance. A flow state occurs when you perfect an action or behavior. It's the goal of maximum performance in anything you do. Athletes strive to reach a flow state so they can win or reach their goal. A laborer achieves maximum productivity when in the flow state. A writer in a state of flow can put words on the page without resistance. The very essence of a professional is the ability to work, create, or perform at the flow state based on positive behavioral habits.

On the contrary, if you let a bad habit like overeating become a flow state, then your maximum performance is adding weight. This is a major cause of the obesity pandemic—most people are efficient at attaining a flow state of sedentary behavior and subconscious eating. They do nothing at maximum performance. They are the best of the best at being sedentary, an expert at overindulging and overeating at maximum efficiency. Yes! You can become an expert in something bad. Once a state of flow is developed for a repeated behavior, the maximum performance of that behavior is almost unavoidable.

From Thought to Product

To summarize, our behaviors originate from thoughts and feelings. When we repeat the same behavior to a response, it becomes routine. When a routine is repeated over time, a habit is developed. When a routine becomes a habit, we can execute the behavior or action without much resistance. Once we execute it enough times, we reach expert-level performance, which leads to maximum performance of behavior. When we execute at maximum performance, we achieve a state of flow over time, with maximum production as the result. Our behavior becomes easy, so easy that we do it subconsciously. This is the basis of reaching a flow state of performance. You're so damn good at it, you can do it without consciously thinking about it.

Let's face it, many of us have become experts at bad behaviors due to routine execution and habit formation. Are you are so good at any bad behaviors or habits that you execute them daily in a state of flow—without thought and resistance? These negative flow state behaviors are the ones you need to eliminate. They are destroying your health, causing you pain, making you fat, ruining your relationships, and keeping you down. Instead, we must create positive flow state behaviors, harnessing their power to eliminate as many negative flow state behaviors as possible.

Simply put, positive flow state behaviors lead to positive outcomes, and negative flow state behaviors lead to negative outcomes. In the end, a person's life can be summed up by how many positive flow state behaviors versus negative flow state behaviors they've accumulated. Things like love versus sin, regret versus satisfaction, positive outcomes versus negative outcomes. Negative flow states lead to negative outcomes or *costs*. Positive flow states lead to positive outcomes or *benefits*. Which way are you tipping the scale of life, toward benefits or costs?

In economics, the formula to calculate reward versus benefit is referred to as the cost-benefit analysis. It is designed to help you make the most financially rewarding choice regarding an investment or business decision, but it can also be used to help you make any decision, such as decisions about purchases, the college you'll attend, your career, vacations, and health. The idea of the cost-benefit analysis is that all decisions should be based on the logical assumption that you desire the most beneficial outcome over the least beneficial and costly outcome. Emotions and feelings aside, the correct choice should always be the most beneficial one.

For example, when choosing a partner, you logically should make this decision based on whether the potential mate has more beneficial than costly qualities in relation to what is best for you and your life. If the results of the cost-benefit analysis are more or higher costs than benefits, then the decision to move forward with this person is an obvious no. And that decision should be made swiftly so you can move on to the next potential partner, one who has a higher benefit over cost ratio. Making choices this way will lead to a life heavy-handed with benefit.

Another law of economics is the law of supply versus demand, which explains that when something in demand becomes limited, its price is high. This limited resource is considered scarce, and scarcity makes it more valuable. Time is scarce and limited. In life, it is usually in later years when we finally become aware of the value of time and its scarcity. So, when making a decision on something important where the costs outweigh the benefits, it does not make sense to waste any more time.

When we choose to eat unhealthy foods, to forgo exercise in lieu of sedentary time, or to avoid medical care, we are making unhealthy choices and ignoring the obvious costs. The costs are the negative outcomes plus the loss of the benefits of making the other choice, such as the lost benefits of receiving medical care. It's a double whammy when you choose the costliest decision because you get the heavy-handed costs and lose all the potential benefits. Over time, all those costly decisions accumulate as negative results, which compound into a life of regret. The costs are your physical, mental, and cognitive health. This is how obesity, type 2 diabetes, smoking, alcoholism, and other unhealthy habits develop. These costly behaviors stack up on each other and progress into more comorbidities, higher disability, and early mortality. Repeatedly making heavy-handed costly choices leads you to become a winner at losing and efficient at failing.

Regret is the outcome of costly choices. The regret may be felt immediately, like a hangover after drinking too much, or over time, like becoming obese or an addict. The opposite of regret is satisfaction.

Jeff Bezos, the founder of Amazon and one of the richest people in the world, tries to live with as little regret as possible so he can have maximum satisfaction in life. He calls this idea *regret minimalization*. When contemplating an investment or decision in life, look ahead to your end-of-life years and imagine how you would feel if you chose or did not choose the path that will end with the least regret. Adapt this mindset for the long term; then in the future, when you are looking back on your life, you will feel satisfied and have no regrets.

Living a life of minimal regret coincides with living a life of the most benefit. Regret is also a cost, which compounded will lead to a life of maximal costs and maximal regret. In the future, a person with a costly and regretful life will look back with anxiety, sadness, and grief. There is no rolling back the hours. No time machine to go back and undo regrettable decisions. Heavy-handed costly decisions lead to regretful results. Cumulative regret leads to failure.

What can you do with this information?

In your journey to maximize your immunity, you must make positive changes that will unfold into the idea of future you. *Future you* is the body you want to be in, the thoughts you want to be thinking, the feelings you want to be feeling, and the satisfaction you will have when you look back on your life. Future you is happy, energetic, strong, enthusiastic about the future, and immune to sickness, disease, disability, and early mortality. Future you is experiencing a body with heavy-handed benefits, no regrets, and maximum immunity. Future you is disciplined and self-confident, someone who attracts positive outcomes from the universe and whose positivity or vibration is contagious. Future you is within your grasp.

Achieving future you starts with your mindset—your CEO. The CEO is driven by what thoughts and underlying emotions are active right now. Focus on your thoughts first. Rather than sleepwalking through life, purposefully think. Repeat your thoughts verbally to set them in stone—a positive affirmation—and make sure that every thought is conducive to achieving future you. Visualize yourself doing what is necessary for change, such as eating lean, exercising, and act on it now! Why wait? In other words, think and grow into future you now, tomorrow, and the next day. Picture yourself as future you at this moment, and do what future you would do to maintain excellence. Your mind will connect to the universe, and with persistence and disciplined maintenance of purposeful thoughts and visualization, future you will become a reality. You will attract all the qualities and benefits that future you entails.

Next, work on your emotions. Rather than reacting to emotions, feel them. Identify whether each emotion is going to hurt or help your outcomes. You want to avoid negative emotions that will lead to regrettable acts or verbalizations, and change them to positive emotions. To do this, you need to learn how to regulate your emotions. Regulating your emotions is as simple as choosing a thought with your power of free will. From our thoughts and emotions, we act. How you act is a product of your behavior. Behaviors or actions that you do repeatedly like eating, sleeping, and practicing self-care become routine. Routine behaviors over time become subconscious and are executed with maximum efficiency. Routines develop into habits. Habitual behaviors over time lead to flow state efficiency. Flow state behaviors are the subconscious actions you have mastered to the point of maximum efficiency. You must eliminate negative flow state behaviors and maximize positive flow state behaviors until they become habitual and eventually positive flow state actions.

Finally, focus on making the most beneficial choices out of *every* decision. Compounding beneficial choices leads to heavy-handed beneficial results and the least cost. Remember, time is a scarce resource, and the time for transformation is now. You cannot undo what was done, but you can do what must be done now. When you weigh the benefits versus costs, think to the future and imagine what choice will carry the most regret looking back on your life. You must make the choice that will result in the least regret possible. Adopt this universal law as a personal law. Starting with your thoughts and emotions, transform yourself through positive behavior modification, routine development, and habit development, and fully harness the productive power of positive flow states. In time, you will win *future you*—and it all starts with a thought that attracts.

Here is a list of what to eliminate from your life, leaving room for positive replacements:

- Negative thoughts
- Negative emotions
- Negative behaviors
- Negative flow state behaviors
- Negative flow state routines
- Negative flow state habits
- Heavy-handed costly choices
- Regret

Think it so, and it will become so.

Visualize it into existence.

Become the CEO you need to be.

CHAPTER SEVEN
THE WORK

Every human is born with a purpose. A purpose changes the world and in death leaves a legacy. Your purpose requires action toward what is necessary to win—to fulfill your purpose. Your win is the reward of your work. Something you do, create, make, innovate, share, transform, influence, or bake is the work of your purpose at the moment. A goal is your vision of the future; your desire to achieve the goal instills purpose, which draws you to action steps that help you reach the goal and thus fulfill your purpose. You need to set goals and draft the action steps, which will lead you to your overall purpose of living—at the moment. Goals and action steps can change in a moment. Without goals, there is no purpose. Without action steps, there is no fulfillment. Find your purpose—fulfill it. In this moment and every consecutive one, get shit done. Now! Not later. Living is now; death is later.

To live on purpose requires both conscious thought and movement toward achieving your goals. On the contrary, living in passivity and without purpose is subconscious living—in other words, *living dead*. The worst-case scenario of living without purpose is subconscious, sedentary behavior, which keeps you from attaining your goals and makes you susceptible to comorbidities. Are you living toward your purpose, or are you living dead?

Work is what keeps all living things alive and vital. Work is necessary; it is the secret sauce of life that helps us find our purpose, attain vitality, find satisfaction, earn longevity, and maintain maximal immunity. Work is an active state of existence. Without work, there is no purpose. Without purpose, you merely exist. Only through active and purposeful work can the mind and body receive the benefits of work.

You cannot make money doing nothing. You cannot produce without first giving something. You do not deserve if you do not contribute. Opposition to this is in opposition to the *law of conservation of mass*, which states during the transfer of matter and energy, mass must remain unchanged over time, and since mass cannot change, matter and energy cannot be created or destroyed. In other words, you can't have *no matter* and *get matter*—a weight or mass of zero will always be zero. Oh, but the cost of nothing—the cost of nothing, which is inaction, is great. The cost of nothing is something that could have been. Inaction makes productivity impossible. Inaction is being passive in this moment, until the next, and so on. Nothing is accomplished in a passive state.

Passivity is submitting to rest; it's the opposite of work. Passivity is living in the subconscious mind, which is absentminded living. Subconscious living is not living at all, it's merely existing and going through the motions.

Do you find yourself just *going through the motions* day by day? If you do, it is time to reinvent yourself. What good is life if you have no good memories of it, no fruits of your labor, no benefit attained or given away? You cannot go back in time and do the work you regret not doing when you were existing subconsciously. Do not avoid doing the work that will benefit you and others. If you have work to be done, it is meant to be done. This is your purpose.

Work provides exercise for the mind and body. Without the stimulus from work, your mind will eventually succumb to early senility, brain atrophy, and dysfunctional thoughts. Without the mental, cognitive, and physical stimulus from work, your body cannot perform efficiently. A muscle without stimuli will atrophy. Bones without stimuli degrade. Organs without stimuli will fail. Maintaining the constant stimuli of work for your body and your mind is key to longevity.

Your spirit also requires work. The work required to fulfill your purpose, mission, and goals gives you satisfaction, self-identity, self-confidence, gratitude, and maximal wellbeing. Work is food for the soul. Doing the work of your mission fulfills your purpose. Being in the service of others is a common path to fulfilling one's purpose in life. Helping others is the ultimate form of personal fulfillment. Like Tony Robbins says, "The secret to living is giving." Most people seek to consume or get, rather than to serve or give. Find work that helps you fulfill your purpose. Living is giving forth and receiving, not merely consuming.

Work is also a way to produce a financial reward. Whether you were born into riches, poverty, or somewhere in between, work remains necessary for survival. You need money to pay for housing, food, water, clothing, utilities, and transportation. You cannot support yourself or others on nothing. Money in your hand is the benefit you receive for your work—or for someone else's work. Government welfare, Medicaid, subsidized housing, food stamps, and other "free lunch" resources are funded with tax dollars. Tax dollars are funds that someone worked for and handed over to the government. If you are dependent on the government for survival, then you are dependent on other working people's earned income. If you are using someone else's money, then you owe a debt. Whether it is a debt of gratitude, of barter or trade, or of repayment, debt has been created and someone, or some entity, now has power and leverage over you.

Financial stress can inhibit your mental, emotional, and physical health, as well as depress your immune system. An example of this is in an article on health.com by Amanda MacMillan and Mia Taylor titled, "7 Ways Debt Is Bad for Your Health." These seven health inhibitors caused by poor financial health and bad debt are:

1. Elevated blood pressure
2. Anxiety
3. Depression
4. Lower immunity
5. Decreased likelihood of going to see a doctor or obtain treatment
6. Higher rates of chronic aches and pains
7. Higher prevalence of ruined relationships

Debt is the opposite of earning the reward for work. Debt is receiving the benefit of work without working, which creates a void. Remember, nothing can come of nothing, and money does not just miraculously appear. Debt can be beneficial for all of us; however, this is only true if it can be successfully fulfilled. Unfulfilled debt contracts, handshake deals, or promises made by intention can lead to some of the highest costly outcomes, stress, ruined relationships, and negativity in life's journey. This negativity leads to stress, which hampers your whole body and mind. Do not accumulate debt unless you can successfully fulfill the obligation to the original owner. Do not seek to be dependent but independent and in control of your life today and as it unfolds tomorrow. In the mission to maximize your health and immunity, you must also manage your finances appropriately.

Work is hunting or gathering food, building or constructing a shelter, fishing, gardening, farming, tending to animals or livestock, shoveling snow, taking out the garbage, clocking in daily at employment, being an entrepreneur, going to school, teaching, or doing infinite other possibilities left to the imagination. So long as you are executing purpose, stimulating your mind, challenging your body, and producing benefits, you are doing a form of work. If you are missing any one of these attributes, the quality of work diminishes.

Stress

Work is a form of stress. There is good stress and bad stress. Good stress stimulates the mind, body, and spirit for the better. Bad stress causes harm. Good stress on the body comes from things like exercise, weight training, chore completion, self-care, walking, running, manual labor, gardening, and being productive at work. Good stress for the mind involves problem-solving, creating, art, writing, puzzles, debating, playing a musical instrument, helping other people, contributing to the community, and planning toward goals. Good stress boosts your immunity.

Emotional stress is bad stress. Negative feelings wreak havoc within the body by releasing cortisol, adrenaline, epinephrine, and other catabolic agents (those that break something down). Emotional stress can lead to a toxic load of anxiety, anger, depression, headaches, worry, weight gain, impaired memory, decreased concentration (the CEO), and harm to the physiological operations of the body, leading to high blood pressure, elevated heart rate, fatigue, digestive problems, poor sleep, heart disease, mitochondrial damage, reduced metabolism, low testosterone, and pain. Bad stress decreases your immune function and makes you susceptible.

Good work stress is positively stimulating for both the mind and the body. If the stress stimulates negative feelings, releases harmful chemicals in the body, or incapacitates your purpose, it is bad work stress. Many people receive bad work stress at their place of employment.

Just as you use the cost-benefit analysis to help you choose benefits over costs and minimize regret, you can use it to minimize negative or bad stress. Just as you must choose the heavy-handed beneficial path, you can choose to forgo any choice that may lead to heavy-handed negative stress. If your place of employment results in heavy-handed negative stress, then it is essential that you decrease the negative stress or find new employment that is heavy-handed in good stress. Work takes up a majority of your life, and life is too short to wallow in negativity.

Unemployment

Employment is work. It's also necessary to earn money. Unemployment is a state of not working and not producing money. You can be unemployed and productive doing things like taking care of the kids, cleaning the house, preparing meals, and doing the yardwork, but none of these productive jobs earn any money. In fact, they use up money. Living consumes valuable resources and money. This is a constant.

Unemployment can lead to financial stress, which is negative stress. Not having enough money to pay the bills, buy groceries, fuel the car, or do fun things leads to overwhelming negative stress. This type of stress can lead to poor health outcomes like anxiety, frustration, depression, low self-esteem, low self-confidence, and other health issues. Long-term unemployment can lead to poverty. When unemployment rises, so does crime. The unemployment rate is also associated with increased divorce rates because long-term socioeconomic hardship erodes marital stability. Alexandra Killewald, a sociology professor at Harvard University, authored a study that found unemployed men are 33 percent more likely to divorce than men who maintain full-time employment.

Unemployment can make you susceptible and sick. According to research reported in a Reuters Health article, the stress caused by unemployment may lower a healthy person's immune system function, increasing their risk of infection and other illnesses. Per a research study done by the University of California, San Francisco, the negative stress from unemployment, which leads to poorer health and lower immunity, *can be undone by getting employed*. According to the study, working again can restore the fighting power of a person's immune system. Work, in particular employment for money, maximizes your immunity by decreasing survival worries and fortifying financial security.

The Body of Work

The health benefits of active work are well documented. Exercise, weight training, manual labor, and other variants of physical resistance all strain the body. The higher level of activity, the higher stress (good stress) on the heart, lungs, cardiovascular system, and every cell in the body. Without continual physical strain, the body succumbs to the effects of sedentary behavior: weakness, deconditioning, sarcopenia, and increased susceptibility to illness, disease, and disability.

Muscles require resistance to stimulate the body and, at a minimum, maintain muscle mass. The phrase *use it or lose it* is true for muscles. If you do not give your muscles regular resistance, your body senses that it doesn't need the muscles and will prune them to the size needed for your lesser physical demands. The result of this process is referred to as *physiological accommodation* and *muscle atrophy*. Muscle atrophy has only negative outcomes unless you like having less power and greater weakness, looking and feeling puny, lowering your metabolism, producing less energy and vitality, reducing your work output, and lowering your immunity. All these consequences lead to greater susceptibility to illness, disease, and disability. Less muscle also makes you more prone to adding body fat and becoming obese.

When you are sick, diseased, in recovery, injured, or experiencing another scenario that results in a high potential for muscle atrophy, it is not the health problem that causes muscle atrophy; it is the sedentary behavior that results from the comorbidity. Whatever the precursor of sedentary behavior, muscle atrophy is due to the lack of manual resistance or work, and it typically corresponds with protein malnutrition too. The best way to counteract muscle atrophy is through routine weight training or another resistive exercise and daily high-quality protein consumption.

Muscles require higher-intensity resistance to trigger muscle tissue growth. The more muscle you have, the stronger you can become. The more resistance you endure, the stronger you condition yourself to be. Metabolic rate corresponds directly to lean body mass, so the more muscle mass you have, the more you can eat without worrying you'll add body fat or become obese.

Research has shown that the immune system is stronger for people with more lean muscle mass. Factors like stress, sleep, and diet also affect the immune system. We have already addressed the importance of eliminating negative stress in attaining maximal immunity. We will address sleep and diet in later chapters.

Hyperactivity

Many people have sedentary jobs. Many people are not employed, whether they're stay-at-home parents, homemakers, retired, seeking education or a job, or disabled. Even if your job is predominantly sedentary, at the least you are forced to get up, get dressed, get in your car, walk into work, walk around some at work, and then return home. If you're a stay-at-home employee, then you have lost the minimum amount of activity provided by an employer-based sedentary job. Supplementing resistive strenuous activity is vital for anyone who has a sedentary job or is unemployed.

The first way to increase your daily activity level is to increase your level of resistance, intensity, and speed, starting with waking up. When you get up, get up! From the moment you are up and running, do everything with a hyperfocus, from self-care to home chores to work. Brush your teeth fast, get dressed fast, walk around fast. Pick things up faster, do the laundry with spunk, and clean the house quickly and with more intensity. The faster you do things, the higher your heart rate, the better your blood circulation, and the more calories you'll use. This will create greater resistance on your body. Day after day, you will have added a great amount of movement and resistance, consumed more energy, and achieved maximal efficiency, resulting in higher overall production.

From human reproduction to what the best of us create, we all benefit from some form of work. Without purpose, without production, without the benefit of work, you are living dead. The foundation of your life can be built stronger with the benefits of work; you are better prepared to help others. Work can be stressful, but heavy-handed positive stress will make you stronger. Therefore, you must make the most beneficial choices to rid your life of negative stress. Nonpurposeful unemployment leads to negative stress, increased susceptibility to health issues, financial distress, and undesired psychosocial outcomes. If you purge negative environments, negative people, and negative benefits from your life, only the positivity remains. Always strive to engage in the production of the show, which is your life. This is your only chance on the stage; we only get one live performance. Continually engaging in active work will keep you healthy, vital, and living with purpose. Remember, always be hyperactive in all you do to maximize the efficiency of your limited time and exceed all outcome expectations, whether yours or those of others.

CHAPTER EIGHT

C.A.R.E

The driving force behind the principles in this book stem from my discovery of the outstanding *preventable* traits of people admitted to the hospital in general. These discoveries are also drawn from my decades of acute care experience and disaster response training in anthrax, severe acute respiratory syndrome (SARS), the bird flu (H5N1), methicillin-resistant Staphylococcus aureus (MRSA), the swine flu, the H1N1 flu pandemic, Ebola, the Zika virus, and the COVID-19 pandemic. And being a Pacific Northwest resident, murder hornets.

To acquire maximum pandemic immunity, you cannot build your pandemic armor on a weak foundation. A weak foundation leaves you susceptible. The integrity of your foundation hinges on the quality of your self-care, your CEO performance, and your ability to work. To help you achieve your best self-care, CEO, and work, I have drawn out a detailed plan of action based on what you can control, take an active stance on, be responsible for, and execute:

C: Control
A: Action
R: Responsibility
E: Execution

The idea behind the C.A.R.E. acronym is that you must do a good job caring for yourself before you can tackle any higher-level skills in your life, like fighting off a predator or dangerous person, moving to safety, building shelter, hunting for food, caring for kids or elders, and contributing to your community. If you're susceptible, weak, and unhealthy, you will not be able to do these things when a pandemic hits; you will be dependent on others.

The outcomes of your life and the quality of your life stem from your ability to execute basic human responsibilities. Your base human condition is a combination of how you care for your body, your ability to choose your thoughts and regulate your emotions, and from there doing the work necessary for your survival, to earn money, to complete goals, and to live with purpose. When you have established a firm foundation in these basic life matters, your probability of success is secured. You'll increase your chance of feeling satisfied with your life, of learning and earning more, and of building your immunity to create powerful, resilient pandemic armor.

"C"
CONTROL

Freedom is control in your own life. —*Willie Nelson*

You control you. Unless you are a child or are mentally, physically, or cognitively disabled, nobody will control you or the outcome of your life. You are stuck with this basic paradigm until your death. The gift of life and with it the right of free will has been yours since birth—with the power of it constrained by your parents, teachers, and mentors until you were deemed a responsible adult.

In the journey of your adult life, there will be mentors, coaches, guides, signs, influence, intuition, and inspiration from the universe to help you succeed and push you to do the right thing—but no one person has power over your control of self. With this power, you can realize your vision of how you want to be—how you want to feel, and how you choose to experience your finite time here on earth.

Most people waste these valuable resources and coast along as the living dead, always hoping to find satisfaction but finding themselves heavy with regret. This is the result of viral irresponsibility and lack of self-control. So many are lost without purpose, crying out in violence and pandemonium about their dissatisfaction and failure to achieve any noticeable significance, complaining about unmet expectations, and trying to justify their unjustifiable complaints, all the while blaming anything and everybody else for their unhappy, unfulfilled lives. The fault in those living in regret, unhappiness, and dissatisfaction is not ours; the fault is all on their shoulders just as yours is on your shoulders. Deflection will not heal your pain . . . *but* if you grab that shit by the horns and fight back with enthusiasm, passion, and purpose, you will ride your eight-second ride.

I am betting that you are taking a stand and are ready to do the work necessary to build yourself up. The mere fact that you are reading this book shows your effort in controlling the results of your life.

Good for you. You just erected a pillar in the foundation of your humanity—it is called *self-care*.

Control over your self-care is the first focus area. Look at all attributes of your self-care, and work on each focus area of the C.A.R.E. acronym until you can be certain that you are in full control over executing maximum-quality self-care at hyperspeed. If you are not living with C.A.R.E., then you have no control over it.

Are you in control of your self-care? Let's go through each act of basic self-care and do a self-assessment to determine just how much control you have.

First is toileting. Toileting involves every step of being able to go to the bathroom—getting on and off a toilet or if outdoors squatting and hovering, managing your clothing, and wiping yourself clean for both bowel and bladder excrement. You need to be able to toilet yourself in the desert, forest, jungle, winter wonderland, or wherever you end up. If you are not in full control over toileting yourself, then you need to fix the problem. Are you in full control over your toileting? Does another person wipe your butt? Do you need to lose weight to be able to reach it? Do you need to start stretching to become more flexible?

The next act is getting yourself dressed. Getting dressed involves being able to put on and take off your undergarments, socks, pants, shirt, and shoes. Are you in full control of getting yourself dressed, or do you avoid getting fully dressed due to difficulty? Do you need someone else to dress you? Do you not wear socks because getting them on is a personal pain point—you're too fat, stiff, or deconditioned?

Bathing involves being able to get naked and use soap and water to thoroughly clean all your body orifices and parts. You need to be able to bathe yourself in a tub, shower, lake, river, or creek, and at minimum give yourself a sponge bath using a pail of water. Are you in full control over your ability to bathe yourself in whatever setting necessary? Do you depend on another person to wash your body? Do you limit yourself to sponge bathing because getting in and out of the tub or shower is too difficult? Have you stopped bathing because it is too difficult? Do you need to lose weight, start exercising, or stretch to reengage in this self-care?

Grooming and oral hygiene is a seemingly easy self-care task, yet I see many people in my practice who cannot do it—so they don't, or they do it with poor quality. They lack control. Are you in control of your ability to brush your teeth, floss, use mouthwash, trim and groom your hair, clean your eyes, shave, trim your nose and ear hairs, put on antiperspirant/deodorant, trim your fingernails and toenails, and care for your skin wounds? If not, then you need to identify the problems and fix them.

What is the performance of your basic mobility? Things like getting in and out of bed, walking around the house, going up and down stairs, getting on and off the toilet, getting in and out of a tub or shower, and getting in and out of a car? If you struggle with any of these basic and necessary movements, you are highly susceptible to failure if pandemonium, catastrophe, or a high-death-rate pathogen hits. If you struggle to move, then there is no way you will be successful running from danger—let alone navigating uneven, elevated, or declined terrain or surviving mother nature's harsh elements. If you are struggling with any tenant of basic mobility, you need to figure out what the problems are and fix them. Your life may depend on it during a regional, national, or global catastrophe.

If you are not in control of any act of self-care, why? If it is your build, then you need to lose weight and trim down to a functional size. If it is weakness, then you need to start a weight training and exercise program. Is the problem lack of muscle mass and protein malnutrition? Then you need to start a resistance training program and eat more meat, fish, and eggs and drink protein shakes. Maybe you can remedy the problem by adapting your environment—like adding a grab bar by your toilet. But your modified environment will be difficult to take with you if a catastrophe has you on the run.

Obesity is due to poor self-control with eating compounded with lack of physical activity. It is a disabling and highly susceptible state. To gain maximum pandemic armor, you must lose your body fat and get down to a healthy thin weight. Fat people cannot run from danger, hide, or fight off danger. They are compromised. There are no fat people alive in the TV series *The Walking Dead*—ever notice that? Fat, deconditioned, and slow people are the first to die when shit hits the fan.

So are sarcopenic people, who also suffer from a highly susceptible and weak state that takes away your control of self. If you lack muscle mass and have protein malnutrition, then you need to start weight training and consuming much higher levels of high biological value/high-quality protein sources to build back your lean muscle mass, power, and stamina.

The combination of obesity and sarcopenia is termed *sarcopenic obesity*. This disabling and feeble state of existence leaves you without control over yourself. A person who is obese with low lean body mass is weak, heavy, and highly susceptible to poor self-care, poor mobility, and illness. They need to start cardiovascular exercise, weight training, fasting, or dieting with high consumption of lean, high biological value protein sources, and other protein supplementation.

A person who smokes anything is susceptible to respiratory dysfunction. Young people will be minimally affected, but as they age, respiratory illness and disease will begin to overtake their performance of self-care, mobility, and fortitude. Moderate to severe respiratory disease results in the inability to walk or run for long enough to survive, let alone manage uphill and downhill terrain or the elements. Having respiratory disease leaves you highly susceptible to other comorbidities, which will further impair your ability to survive a catastrophe. Quit smoking everything—it is that simple. There is no other way. Smoking or not smoking is all about control over yourself.

Substance addiction incapacitates a person's judgment, personal motivations, and overall survivability. The older the addict becomes, the higher the susceptibility to illness and disease, and the greater the inability to run, hide, fight back, or survive the elements, predators, or disease. Quit drinking alcohol or minimize its consumption. Quit doing drugs—it is that simple. There is no other way. Control yourself.

Let's face it. If the world goes to shit because of a catastrophic highly contagious pathogen, a zombie virus, a war on home ground, global anarchy and rioting, an alien invasion, or an event horizon, if you can't self-care, do your chores, manage survival protocols, walk, run, drive, hide, or quarantine, then your chances of surviving are low. If you have to depend on others because you cannot self-care and do the work required for survival, then you are unprepared for catastrophe. Because you are not in control, you will die when no one is able or willing to wipe your butt, do your chores, hunt, farm for your food, or fight for your survival.

Control can only be attained with the proper mindset. Your thoughts must support your self-care and self-sufficiency in all aspects of life's responsibilities. You must think you can self-care, do your chores, survive, and do whatever else is necessary to repair, remediate, or rehabilitate any deficits in your ADL, IADL, and work function.

Harnessing control over attributes of yourself will take work. This may mean exercising, weight training, staying disciplined in a restrictive diet to lose weight, or seeking someone outside yourself—mentorship, coaching, therapy, or personal training—to help you be successful.

Chaos

The opposing force of control is chaos. If you are not in control, you are in chaos. Chaos leads to unpredictable behaviors and outcomes, disorder and confusion, disorganization, and failure. Prevent pandemonium in your life and increase your chances of survival by maintaining control

"A"
ACTION

Action is the foundational key to all success. —Pablo Picasso

Action gets things done. Only through action can you change. Action is movement of your body, conscious use of your mind for purposeful thought. Action stimulates your mind and body. The muscles of your body need action to thrive.

Self-care is in fact action in motion. "Action," the director yells out, then the cameras roll film, and the act begins. You are the actor in the performance of your life. Imagine you are dead and are able to look at your life in its entirety—at your life's performance. How was your stage performance here on earth? Did you put on a good show, performing at your maximum potential, or did you put on a cheap, low-quality performance with minimal benefit to the world? How you act out your life and the sequence of events in it are your show—your performance. If you are not acting it out, then there will be no production—no performance to observe or benefit from. For example, an obese, sedentary person fails to act out their purpose in life by spending their days in a recliner, eating and binge-watching TV shows, movies, and social media. This show is boring. This person has no product; rather, they consume, which leaves them susceptible to sickness, disease, disability, and death during a pandemic.

A successful performance takes disciplined practice, purposeful thought, and enthusiastic execution of your talent. This acting concept is necessary for all important aspects of your life, including relationships, employment, and your community.

You will be judged by and rewarded for your performance. If your acting blows—if the results of your actions suck—so will the reward and recognition you receive in return. The act you deliver to the universe will come right back at you the same.

Your thoughts must proclaim action. They must be detailed, purposeful, and executional. You are the CEO, and everything hinges on your action-driven mindset. Many scenes or performances take multiple attempts to get them right; that's why the director yells out, "Take one!" "Take two!" "Take three!" Likewise, some acts in the performance of your life will take multiple attempts before being successfully done. Out of repeated failures comes the successful final act. Then it's on to the next act in your life performance.

Work is action. Action is work. Both require physical output and skilled or critical thinking, ultimately fulfilling a purpose. You must do the work; you must take action and do it with maximum conviction. Anything less will peter out and result in low production.

Apathy

The opposing force to action is apathy. Apathy is a lack of ambition and responsiveness in thoughts, behaviors, feelings, actions, and work. The lack of desire apathetic people feel is due to their underlying comorbidities, unhappiness with themselves, and low self-confidence. To resolve apathy, first focus on maximizing self-care, then on the performance of your act. Finally, do the work, and do it with enthusiasm.

"R"

RESPONSIBILITY

You cannot escape the responsibility of tomorrow by evading it today. —Abraham Lincoln

No one is responsible for you. It is all on you—your education, training, career, relationships, car, house, and the quality of it all. Everything you yearn for is in the air you breathe. But it's your responsibility to get. The good life is not given; it is earned. So long as you are living, you can achieve.

Self-care is a personal responsibility. Your mommy is not there to wipe your nose, brush your teeth, and remind you to shower. It is your job to take care of your body and your mental health, so just frickin' do it!

Your soiled laundry, your unclean and cluttered home, your sullied car, and your messy work desk are the product of your doing—your incomplete responsibilities. The product and the results of your work hinge on the quality of your IADL. Do your laundry and wear clean clothes, tidy up your house and get rid of shit you don't need, clean out and wash your car, and declutter your desk. I'm sorry to break it to you, but nobody gives a flying hoot about you and your responsibilities—and whether or not you take care of business. Every other person on this earth, including your friends, family, and loved ones, has their own responsibilities; no one has a surplus of energy or time to worry about yours. You need to worry about yourself and take care of your problems, your self-care, your chores, your work, and your responsibilities.

What are you thinking? Do you believe in yourself and your responsibilities? Hopefully, you do because nobody else does. Be the responsible CEO of your life. Think and self-care. Think and do your chores. Think and do the work. Think and believe in yourself. Think and be responsible.

When you work, you are taking responsibility for managing your finances, housing yourself, feeding yourself, and growing your wealth. It is your responsibility to do the work that contributes to the universe, your team, your community, and society. The legacy you leave is your responsibility to build.

Refusal

The opposing force to personal responsibility is refusal. Refusal to participate. Denial of your purpose. Refuse responsibility, and you'll pay the price of living irresponsibly: low self-esteem, poor self-confidence, poor decision-making, mistakes, and failure to fulfill your purpose—to have a meaningful life. You will have no pandemic armor if you refuse to do what is necessary to get it—to self-care, finish chores, and engage in productive work.

"E"
EXECUTION

Go get some! —Jocko Willink

The outcomes of your life depend on executing the steps toward your purpose. Nobody else will execute for you. Someone who cares may kick you in the ass, tell you what to do, or attempt to persuade you to execute, but only you can do it.

Step completion, reaching goals, and satisfying your purpose are yours to execute. If you want to be healthy and have maximum immunity, then you must do what is necessary to achieve just that.

If you don't execute and leave the starting line when the race official blasts "Go!" over the loudspeaker, you just lost the race. You may have been physically present, but you weren't emotionally or mentally in the race and stand zero chance of winning, let alone placing. You had no balls. No confidence. Lack of bravery. Lack of willpower. If you want to win the race, you must engage. As engagement intensifies, inertia grows, momentum and power intensify, production becomes evident, and your actions garner results.

To think purposefully first takes desire. If you have no desire, you will not engage, and you will be left with the path of least resistance, destined to live subconsciously. You'll be living in passivity as one of the living dead.

Execute purposeful, positive thoughts, conjure desire from within your soul, and the desire and thoughts you engage in will grow into reality—the vision of future you. Think and be a starter.

Do the work! Get up and get to it. This is how you execute your plan to self-care with quality, to do your chores, to produce for your employer, and to live out your purpose, your passion—and then you win. Your pandemic armor will not build itself, and the more you procrastinate, the more susceptible you remain. Get ready for it. Something bad is always coming, whether pathogens or some other danger, but you can be ready to the best of your ability if you prepare.

Ejection

The opposing force to execution is ejection. You are going to either execute your plan or eject yourself from engagement. Ejection is a false start. If you eject yourself from the race of life, you have no chance to win. Regret is all that remains.

Now that you know how to C.A.R.E., you can build a solid foundation of health, wellness, and work. The need to be in control of yourself, to take action, to harness personal responsibility, and to execute your plan is the foundation of your immunity. The enemy of C.A.R.E. is a life of chaos, apathy, refusal, and ejection, each of which prevents you from acting out your purpose, gaining your health, and being satisfied with your life.

It is time to build your armor for maximum immunity. You do not want to be one of the susceptible dying in the hospital from the next global pathogen. You do not want to be part of the Obesiboomer generations living with massive susceptibility, comorbidities, disease, and disability. You do not want to end up wallowing in a state of poor quality of life—all because you did not care for yourself, take action in your life, and do the work when you could have done it. You do not want to die early. Fight to live.

You want health.

You want longevity.

You want function and independence from others.

You want to follow your passion and live out your purpose.

You want to be prepared for the next pandemic, natural catastrophe, or zombie apocalypse.

You are willing to do the work.

You are going to take a stand.

You are ready to "go get some!"

You are ready to build your armor.

And I have created a plan for you to achieve it. The C.A.R.E. solution is the foundation for your A.R.M.O.R.

Before we explore the plan for building your A.R.M.O.R., let's go through a few case studies to help secure your understanding of how to execute the C.A.R.E. solution.

Dadbod David

David grew up in Tennessee with four younger siblings and his single mother. He did not attend higher-level education, and most of his training on self-care, personal responsibility, and work was taught to him by a few sparingly attentive public-school teachers and his mother, who worked two jobs and divided her attention among work, home, and five needy kids. David did much of his own self-learning, behavior and habit formation, and planning for adulthood. No trust fund, no college money, no external family support. He was basically on his own. It was just how the cards were dealt for David.

He is now forty-two years old and married with three kids. He has a body mass index (BMI) of 36 and a growing potbelly to boot. He gets short of breath when he tries to play with his kids, sports, or physical activities. He works as a dispatcher for the local public utility, which provides him a decent income, a health plan, and retirement benefits. He enjoys his job and plans to retire when he turns sixty-five.

Everything seems pretty well off for David, but what you see on the surface is not the full story. David is having marital problems. His wife has grown distant from David. She is frustrated with the burden of chores and her stay-at-home-parent situation, as well as with David.

Their marital problems stem from three very important aspects that are easily *preventable*. The first is that David has been dealing with erectile dysfunction for about two years now. This has led to poor self-confidence, negative thoughts, and for the most part, avoiding any attempts to be intimate with his wife. The second is that because of David's upbringing and lack of good mentorship or parenting, he failed to adopt the importance of good personal hygiene and personal ownership of chores. His mom did it all, so he learned not to do it at all. And the third problem is that David doesn't do a good job washing his body when he showers, even though he showers daily. This leaves him smelling at times, which offends his wife. She has hinted about it many times, and she avoids him because of it. If David does not fix these three simple problems, his marriage will likely end in divorce, and his life will go down the shitter.

David decides to gain control over his life.

David has finally decided that he wants to save his marriage and is willing to do whatever is necessary to make this happen. He has identified the three problems he needs to fix that will likely change his life. He has found a meaningful purpose: to heal his relationship with his wife.

David takes *action*.

He makes an appointment with his doctor about his erectile dysfunction and body odor. In this appointment, he finds out that the main contributing factor of his erectile dysfunction is obesity. (Obesity is a significant risk factor for erectile dysfunction according to PubMed. gov.) He also learns from his doctor that obesity increases difficulty with personal hygiene and gets a referral to see an occupational therapist. David's dadbod is the culprit for much of his health issues, difficulty with self-care, and sexual dysfunction. David has gained a lot of body fat in the last ten years due to his sedentary behavior, sedentary job, and inattentiveness to his diet.

To tackle the problem of erectile dysfunction, rather than resort to boner pills, David gets a gym membership and hires a personal trainer. His trainer helps him create a goal-oriented plan to lose all the body fat, get lean and stronger, and maximize his activity tolerance and endurance. Instead of receiving the benefits of sedentary behavior and inattentive overeating, he will now receive the benefits of exercise, increased activity, and a restrictive and nutritious diet plan.

To tackle his occasional body odor, he sets an appointment with an occupational therapist.

As far as helping out with chores, he decides he needs to sit down with his wife to discuss his health issues, plan of action, and goals. He has asked his wife to help him learn how to vacuum, do laundry, and use the dishwasher. She is pleased.

David is taking responsibility for his health, his body composition, his self-care, his level of activity engagement, his relationship with his wife, and his contribution to the home chores.

To be successful in his transformation goals that his trainer helped him set, David will need to maintain discipline with the workout and diet plan, stay focused on his overall goals using conscious thoughts, maintain a positive mindset (his CEO), and execute his workouts and food restriction with enthusiasm and purpose. These three things— conscious focus, motivation, and positivity—will keep the momentum for change going and help David stay on track for the long term.

In the meeting with the occupational therapist, they identify together David's difficulty with self-care, specifically with bathing, toileting, grooming, and hygiene. The occupational therapy assessment found that based on the size of David's belly, buttocks, and adipose tissue folds compared to his shoulder range of motion, arm length, and overall flexibility, he was struggling to reach all his body parts. The OT educated and trained David on how to thoroughly bathe his upper and lower body, perform quality total-body hygiene self-care using adaptive and modified techniques, and demonstrated a long-handled bath brush for helping him clean hard-to-reach areas of his body. They reviewed how to apply antiperspirant/deodorant, lotion, and cologne. The OT also recommended that for David to achieve long-term self-care independence and maximal quality of life, he should consider treating his obesity—the direct cause of most of his hygiene problems. David explains that he has already identified a plan of action for losing weight and getting in shape with his trainer, which should, in time, improve his ability to reach all areas of his body for bathing and personal hygiene.

Now with plans to extinguish erectile dysfunction, obesity, body odor, and laziness at home, David is ready to execute the steps as prescribed by his doctor, personal trainer, occupational therapist, and wife. David is ready and enthusiastic to complete the necessary work to achieve his goals—to win. He has all the ingredients of C.A.R.E. to fulfill his purpose.

He is taking **control** of his life.

He is taking **action** to find help, make a plan, and do the work.

He is taking personal **responsibility** for his problems.

He is **executing** the plan of action.

One month later, David has lost fifteen pounds and gained two pounds of muscle. He has stopped eating unhealthy, sugary, fattening hyperpalatable foods, alcohol, and snacks. Daily exercise and intermittent weight training are improving his strength, stamina, and overall health. He is noticing that he is feeling better overall, and with that, his libido is returning. With his reduced body mass, his reachability is improving and thus the quality of his personal hygiene and bathing. With his wife's help, he has learned how to do the laundry, which he does whenever he can. He also has learned how to run the dishwasher and do the dishes, which he does daily. He vacuums the house every Saturday. David's wife is noticing everything and is pleased. Her stress is down, so she is happier and leaning more into David. David's personal transformation is obvious and has inspired his wife to exercise more and eat better. David's positive changes are also inspiring to everyone at work. David and his wife are now seeing eye to eye and are working together to improve their relationship. Everything that was ruining David's life is disappearing. So long as David continues with his healthy positive regimen, his life will only get better from here.

Tina TV

Tina loves to watch television and movies. Who doesn't, right? Especially with the addictive nature of TV shows, cliffhanger endings, and ability to watch episodes back-to-back with no advertisements or commercials. Tina will sit for hours straight without getting up unless she needs to reload her snack bowl or use the bathroom. Tina also enjoys reading when she is not watching TV.

She is thirty-six years old, single, and lives alone in a ground-floor apartment. Tina is not working and is being supported by state disability payments. Her inability to work stems from complications with type 2 diabetes and its management. Tina also weighs 235 pounds. She last worked a year and a half ago for a local grocery store as a checker. She enjoyed working and the social interaction with coworkers and customers that came with it. She now finds herself feeling lonely and misses the benefits of work and human interaction. She lives an extremely sedentary existence and does not get out of her apartment much. She is not happy unless she is watching TV and eating.

About three weeks ago, Tina noticed she was starting to lose feeling in her feet. They are getting a little numb and tingly, and she is worried about it. Tina makes an appointment with her doctor.

The doctor tells her that her feet going numb is peripheral neuropathy, irreversible nerve damage caused by her diabetes and poor blood sugar management. She begins to cry, realizing that she will never get her full sensation back in her feet. The doctor also informs her that it will only get worse if she continues to live as she is. The doctor tells her that peripheral neuropathy is a precursor to diabetic skin ulcers, which are wounds that have poor healing because of diabetes, and furthermore, that diabetic ulcers lead to amputation of body parts, usually starting with the toes, then the foot, then below-the-knee and finally above-the-knee amputations.

In shock, Tina asks the doctor if there is anything she can do to prevent her peripheral neuropathy from worsening and the subsequent comorbidities caused by diabetes. The doctor lays it out to her: the number one cause of type 2 diabetes is obesity. Tina needs to lose over a hundred pounds to get down to a healthy normal weight, needs to exercise daily, and needs to adopt healthy eating habits. This plan of action will cure her of obesity and will likely also cure her type 2 diabetes, or at a minimum make it much easier to manage. The doctor refers her for consultation with a diabetes educator, a nutritionist, and a physical therapist (PT).

The diabetes educator teaches Tina how to manage her blood sugars and gives her some tips on weight loss. The nutritionist teaches Tina about the science of fats, proteins, and carbohydrates in general and in particular in dealing with obesity and diabetes. Tina is prescribed a diabetic and weight loss diet plan. The nutritionist will be available by phone, email, and text messaging if Tina has questions along her weight loss journey. The PT assessment reveals that Tina is also dealing with moderate deconditioning and gets short of breath easily with exertional activity; she has to take many breaks to catch her breath going up and down one flight of stairs. Tina is advised to work with the PT for two visits a week for six weeks to condition her until she can take over independently at home or at a community fitness center.

Tina takes the advice of the diabetic educator and nutritionist and goes to the grocery store to stock up on lean fish, chicken breasts, whey protein powder, vitamins, fibrous vegetables, and other diabetic- and low-calorie-approved foods. Her diet will consist mostly of lean meats, protein shakes, and low-calorie, low-glycemic carbohydrates. (*Glycemic* refers to how a carbohydrate affects a person's blood sugar. The higher the glycemic rating, the more the carbohydrate raises blood sugar levels, and the lower the rating, the lower the blood sugar response.) Tina will also stop all snacking and cut back on sedentary time. She plans to replace time watching TV and movies with going on walks to burn calories, improving her endurance and strength with the goal of being able to go hiking in the mountains someday.

At her physical therapy sessions, she learns how to use a treadmill and an elliptical trainer. She progresses the duration and resistance levels incrementally on the stair climber. She progressively increases the resistance each weight training session, leading to strength gains. For all exercises in general, she slowly and strategically taxes her body further. She does not miss any PT appointments and is staying focused on her goal to lose a hundred pounds, get rid of her diabetes, and someday hike up a mountain.

Six weeks have passed, and Tina has completed her physical therapy. The PT has recommended that she get a gym membership and continue to work on her strengthening, endurance, and weight loss plan. In the last six weeks, Tina has lost twenty-two pounds of body fat and gained two pounds of new muscle. She can climb up and down six flights of stairs at a steady pace without taking breaks, walk briskly on a treadmill for twenty minutes on a 3 percent incline, and do ten pounds of resistance training with dumbbells, up from two pounds when she started. She finds herself laughing more, interacting more with people since first seeing her doctor, and having more energy than she can remember having since she was a kid.

Tina has a follow-up appointment with her doctor today. After checking her vitals, blood composition, and body weight, the doctor presents her with great news. "Tina, whatever you are doing, keep doing it! At the rate you're transforming your body, your lab results point toward a resolution of your type 2 diabetes. Good job." A tear falls from the corner of Tina's eye. "Thank you."

Tina underwent a C.A.R.E. transformation. She took **control** by making a doctor's appointment. She took **action** when she went to the doctor, diabetic educator, nutritionist, and PT, and she took action again on their advice and recommendations. She took **responsibility** for her body weight, behavior, activity, diabetes, and diet. She has been **executing** and will continue to execute her daily walks, resistance training at a gym, diet, and socialization with people she meets at the gym and on her walks.

After one year of disciplined execution of her new habits, she has lost over sixty pounds and no longer meets the diagnostic criteria for type 2 diabetes. Thus, she has cured herself by taking care of herself. After climbing to the top of Mount Stuart, she looks up at the sky, hands in the air, and in blissful excitement screams, "What's next?" The next day, Tina turns in an application for employment at a local grocery store.

Greg the Gamer

Greg is twenty-six years old, spends most of his time in the world of online computer gaming, and lives in his younger sister's basement. He is about forty pounds overweight, and other than light activity at work, he is driving in his car or playing video games, both sedentary time. He hates his full-time job at a fast-food establishment. At work, he deals with high-stress customer service, a condescending boss, and a boring thirty-minute commute each way. Greg's sister told him that she is moving in three months and that he needs to get his own place. The negative stress is stacking up on Greg, and he is sick and tired of dealing with it all.

Greg's load of heavy-handed negative benefits stems from his daily behavior and actions. He is reaping what he is sowing. Greg realizes this after he reads the book *EXERLEAN*, which teaches people how to take control of their lives, find purpose, exercise, and eat lean to achieve optimal health, wellness, and productivity as well as peace of mind—which is exactly what he needs to make a whole-life transformation. He learns about the cost-benefit analysis and applies it to his life, weighing the benefits and costs of his actions. He realizes that he has been living a life of heavy-handed negative decisions, weighed with indolent behavior and low productivity, which has led him to regret and dissatisfaction. He becomes inspired to make some drastic changes in his life, including his health and his employment.

Greg has figured out that an abundance of sedentary time and thoughtless eating has led to his weight gain. This sedentary behavior and weight gain have also made him feel deconditioned with low energy. Reading that daily exercise, weight training, and a purposeful diet will help improve his mood, level of happiness, energy, and strength—coincidently through the body's natural release of endorphins and receiving the benefits of exercise and weight training—he decides to go all in. He makes a resolution to achieve a positive life transformation that will change his body composition, his performance, and his mental health, and hopefully help him find a better job.

He visualizes what he wants his life to be like in the future. He pictures himself with forty pounds less body fat and five pounds of newly built muscle. He envisions himself with increased energy and strength to boot. He sees himself living independently in his own residence. He sees himself managing his time better and being more active, working, and still enjoying computer gaming, but less frequently. In the future, he demands happiness and contentment. He aims to stand someday with the least amount of regret and maximal satisfaction with himself and his life.

Greg makes a plan that is approachable, executable, realistic, and entailed with actionable steps, which will unfold into reality, his vision of future him. To manifest his plan, he must reach his goals:

1. Lose forty pounds of body fat through diet and exercise.
2. Add five pounds of lean muscle mass, improve strength, and increase energy for daily activities.
3. Get a better job that will be enjoyable, rewarding, and less stressful.
4. Move into a new place and live independently.

To achieve his goals, he will need to break them up into smaller steps. For the first and second goals, Greg gets a gym membership and makes an appointment with a personal trainer to establish a workout routine and get familiar with the gym. His workout plan involves four days a week of weight training and seven days a week of cardiovascular exercise.

For Greg's third goal, he identifies what makes him unhappy with his job: the long, boring commute, the relationship with his boss, and the stress of fast-paced customer service.

After much thought, Greg decides he wants to find a job that has less face-to-face customer service and more outdoor activity. He applies for a truck-washing position at the local garbage company. He sees this as a great opportunity and a position with possibility for advancement to becoming a garbage truck driver, which will bring with it more physical activity, less customer interaction, and minimal interaction with management throughout the day. The truck-washing job pays more than his current job and in time has the potential for progressively increasing compensation if he earns it. He is called in for an interview and is offered the job. He gives two weeks' notice at the fast-food joint.

He starts looking online and finds an apartment about thirty-five minutes from where his new job will be. The commute will be a little longer, but he cannot find anything closer that he can afford. To make the commute more enjoyable, he loads his cell phone up with audiobooks on self-help, business, and investing so he can continue to improve his mindset, intelligence, and motivation.

Three months later, Greg has accomplished all four of his goals and is now living in the future reality of his past vision. He completed one cardio session a day for a total of ninety cardio sessions. He weightlifted four times a week for a total of forty-eight workouts. He has lost forty pounds of body fat and gained five pounds of new muscle. He is leaner and stronger and feels more energetic. He maintained a high-protein, low-fat, low-carb diet for ninety days without cheating, which set the stage for burning body fat not only during his cardio and weight-training sessions but also throughout the day. During his commute, he averaged one audiobook a week for a total of twelve self-help and educational books—all new knowledge that has inspired him to visualize new goals and continue improving his life. His ninety-day probation period at work is over, and in a follow-up meeting with the boss, he finds out that management has noticed his hard work ethic and his motivation for advancement.

Greg has made great positive changes to his physical health and wellness, his career health, and his mindset through his commute. Greg decided to C.A.R.E. for himself and make positive changes to transform his life. To do this, he first took *control* of his life. He decided that he was in control of finding a new living situation, finding job satisfaction, and improving his physical health and body composition. To take control of his paradigm, he took the necessary *actions* for initiating weight training and exercise at the gym, searching and applying for the truck-washer position, eating more restrictively, and moving to a new place. Greg was able to do all this because he harnessed the power of personal *responsibility* for his situation. Greg completed the actions of his plan, step-by-step, until he *executed* his plan of achieving his vision of his future self.

Anybody can make their lives radically better by first taking control over all aspects of their life paradigm. When you do this, a paradigm shift becomes inevitable.

Only you control you and the outcomes of your life. So long as you are willing and take action by completing the day-by-day steps that lead to your goals, you will achieve transformation. By taking personal responsibility for your health, wellness, and body composition, in time, you can achieve anything you believe you can achieve. Finally, you must do the work. You must execute each step of your plan with enthusiasm and focus. If you do this relentlessly, you will win, and C.A.R.E. will be your foundation for further success and growth.

People stay the same. Day in and day out, they resist change. They live with undesirable stress and choose to continue enduring naysayers, pessimists, toxic work environments, and personal dissatisfaction. This is the way it is because they do not believe they can change, fear the results of change, feel that change will be too difficult, or merely lack the willpower. Shifting your paradigm, whether radically executed or gradual, is not as difficult as it may seem. In fact, the basis for all personal transformation is simple. Getting in better shape is simple. Finding a new job is just a matter of doing it. Enduring negative external influence can be countered with speaking up for yourself. The difficult part of change is always the initial commitment. Once you commit, you can achieve anything. So long as you can envision yourself being different, it can become so. You can achieve the vision of how you want to be, immune with pandemic armor and all.

MAXIMUM IMMUNITY

CHAPTER NINE
A.R.M.O.R.

What is armor?
According to *Merriam-Webster's Dictionary*, armor is:

defensive covering for the body
a quality or circumstance that affords protection
a protective outer layer

There are several examples of armor in nature. The alligator gar is a fish covered in flexible scaled armor that has the texture of teeth. The gar's armor is so strong a knife can't penetrate it. Another animal born with armor is the turtle. A turtle has a thick, almost indestructible shell of armor able to withstand two hundred times its body weight and thousands of pounds of pressure before giving in and crushing—all to protect its owner from predators and the weather. The armadillo has almost bulletproof scaly armor and is the only animal that can roll into a ball of armor for defense. Most insects have a hard exoskeleton that is designed to protect their vulnerable insides. Most animals have some sort of exterior armor like thick skin, coarse hair or dense fur, thick calloused padding, scales, or feathers. So, what is the case for *human* armor?

Specific situations often dictate the form of armor that humans may require. For example, a tank is an armored vehicle designed to withstand the impact of bullets, missiles, and bombs, therefore protecting troops in battle or in transport. Your personal vehicle is a form of armor when you are involved in an automobile accident. A bike helmet is armor for your skull; a skull is armor for your brain. The police wear bulletproof vests and tactical gear for extra protection. This kind of armor would be very expensive, heavy, uncomfortable, and unrealistic to wear for everyday use. In medieval times, a knight wore a metal suit of armor. But today, it's not like you can go to the mall and shop for the newest shiny suit of armor, a new metal helmet, or a big shiny shield with your family crest stamped in gold. Nor would you necessarily need to.

For us everyday Janes and Joes, what are our armor options? On the exterior, it would be our clothing, shoes, gloves, hats, and sunglasses. The thicker and tougher the clothing and outerwear, the higher the protection. But underneath all the polyester and plastic is our most valuable layer of armor—our skin. Our outer skin layer, the epidermis, is the final external protective layer of armor. Everything underneath our skin—fat, muscle tissue, arteries, veins, nerves, blood and other body fluids, connective tissues, and organs are highly susceptible to infection if they come into contact with the exterior world. Outside the epidermis is a cornucopia of bacterial, viral, prion, and unidentified contamination. Our skin is not tough alone. Our skin is thin, giving, and easy to penetrate. For this reason alone, humans are drawn to wearing clothing. Clothing is an extra layer of protection from the sun, pathogens, harsh weather conditions, and predators.

It could be said that any form of armor, from medieval chainmail to a scuba suit to clothes, is designed to protect us from whatever environment we are in and the predators or pathogens living there. The dictionary definition of armor describes it in the realm of the external, but this is incomplete. We are susceptible to airborne, vapor, or droplet pathogens through our natural portals of entry: our nose, mouth, ears, vagina, urethra, and anus. For these unprotected orifices, we have only one line of defense—the immune system.

Our immune system lies underneath the exterior armor and is the most treasured protection system that our body has against the next killer pandemic. This is the last defensive stand of the body. If our exterior armor fails us and we sustain an injury that penetrates our skin, we are then susceptible to infection. If we ingest a pathogen through one of our *always-existing* portals of entry, then we can succumb to illness. At this point, whatever metal, leather, or bulletproof exterior armor you're wearing will not matter. Whether an infection from a wound or a pathogen through another portal of entry, it is all on our immune system to kill off the infecting force and return us to our baseline state.

Your pandemic armor includes both your external and internal elements. The combined strength of your external protection and internal immunity is the full force of your pandemic armor. Your armor is everything you protect your body with when you engage in the world around you. Your immune system is waiting at the ready when your external armor fails you. You must decide just how resilient and strong your armor will be. This is all on you.

We learned in the last chapter that to build up your pandemic armor to a state of maximum immunity, you need a solid foundation. The foundation is built on good self-care, positive thoughts and emotions, and active engagement in ADL, IADL, work, and your purpose. The process of C.A.R.E. will help you eliminate your comorbidities, which leave you susceptible. Caring for yourself will help you to gain control over your thoughts, your body, your health, and your work. The action you are taking will help you transform your life and your production, and it will throw you into the act of living out your purpose. Taking responsibility for yourself, your predicament, and your future leads you to maximum pandemic armor. Your ability to execute a plan that will help you achieve the goals of your purpose and your passion will result in the maximum benefit and the least amount of regret.

The C.A.R.E. process will take time. Eliminating certain comorbidities may be instantaneous, or it may take days, months, or years depending on the comorbidity and its severity. Smoking, doing drugs, or abusing alcohol can be eliminated immediately. In fact, at this very damn moment. Just don't ever pull another cigarette or joint, and from this moment forward, don't take another sip of alcohol. Getting in the habit of performing daily, high-quality self-care can take days to months, and in time you will fully break yourself of poor self-care habits. A dirty house, a filthy car, and a disorganized work desk will take only days to resolve; just get it done. On the other hand, diabetes, heart disease, and obesity will take months to years to eliminate or get under control. Protein malnutrition and muscle atrophy will take months to years to recuperate from because you need to restore the lean mass you lost. How long it takes is not what you should worry about. What matters is that you have a plan to eliminate poor self-care, poor ADL and IADL, sedentary behavior, lack of production and work, and protein malnutrition, and that you take personal action—that you execute your plan! In time, you will achieve all your goals so long as you move progressively toward them. Taking progressive actions over time is the key to success, and your incremental steps toward improvement—even if they're tiny— will compound and eventually deliver you to your envisioned goal. Future you is on the horizon!

You do not have to wait to build your A.R.M.O.R. while you work on your C.A.R.E. foundation. The process of C.A.R.E. will help you build your armor just as the process of A.R.M.O.R. will help you complete the goals of C.A.R.E. The two support one another. What matters most is that you start now, make a plan to achieve maximum immunity, execute your plan, and take action, completing step by step, hour by hour, day by day, week after week, month after month, until your pandemic armor is at the ready. When you have reached maximum immunity, you will need to maintain the thoughts, feelings, behaviors, and actions that get you there. This will ensure maximum longevity and the ability to thrive through whatever negative forces come at you throughout your life.

I have created the A.R.M.O.R. acronym as a guide to help you get your pandemic armor. All the benefits of A.R.M.O.R. are doable, achievable, and receivable. If you follow each step of the plan, take personal responsibility, take action, execute daily, visualize your success, and focus on the goal, you will have your armor.

It is important to understand that all the action steps and protocols in this book are 100 percent attainable. Not only is this all attainable, but it is also simple to transform your subconscious and absentminded thinking, which created your harmful habits, to a conscious and pur-poseful mindset that allows you to live with a positive self-help focus and execute healthy actions, which will help you uninstall deep-seated harmful habits. Everything from having a lean, muscular, strong, enduring, healthy, and immune body, with a super-ready CEO, is going to be your reality so long as you do as instructed.

Herein lies the beginning of your journey to maximize your pandemic armor.

Each letter of A.R.M.O.R. signifies a specific personal trait, behavior, or action step that will maximize your immunity:

A: Activity
R: Rest and Recovery
M: Moderation
O: Obliteration
R: Resolution

Each area of focus provides the necessary information to help you first learn, then do. Every little thing you do to improve yourself will move you down your path to maximum immunity and the development of your pandemic armor.

"A"
ACTIVITY

Physical fitness is not only one of the most important keys to a healthy body; it is the basis of dynamic and creative intellectual activity. —John F. Kennedy

Activity is where armor begins. It is the most important factor in determining your overall health. You know now that sedentary behavior leads to deconditioning, muscle atrophy, lower metabolism, and obesity, all comorbidities that make you susceptible to disease, illness, and infection. The human body is not designed to be in a state of stillness. The body is built with muscles, tendons, and nerves to innovate those muscles—to work, to resist, and to move the body. The heart, arteries, and veins are built to pump, circulate, and transport fuel and nutrients to every cell in the body through the bloodstream. Body fat is beneficial for emergency energy if you're in a state of starvation, which in modern society is almost unheard of. Food is abundant in the world—too abundant in developed countries. The majority of the world's citizens, which have daily access to an infinite amount of food, are coincidently overnourished to the point of disease. Body fat is the epitome of sedentary behavior and overeating. The hood ornament on a glutinous Rolls-Royce. The bulbous gift wrapping and bubble packing on an unhealthy present.

Considering that over 72 percent of Americans are overweight or obese, there is a desperate need for immediate change for the majority. In fact, this change is necessary for most human beings. Obesity is a global problem. Even Japan, the seemingly most healthy nation on earth and well known for the longevity of its people, is becoming obese. The change this world needs involves a multifaceted process that addresses the two main contributors to obesity: sedentary behavior over time and repetitively overeating the wrong foods.

The fact is, a person is either getting fatter, maintaining, or getting leaner. As far as behavior, they are either sedentary or active. Considering that 72 percent of us are overweight or obese, it is logical to assume that the overwhelming majority of us are in a constant state of getting fatter at varying speeds, and that the predominant behavior is to be sedentary. The maintainers are routinely active enough and eat at just the right level to avoid weight gain, but most people who believe they are maintaining are slowly getting fatter, numb to the trickle gains of body fat until it is obesingly apparent later in life and negative health rears its ugly soul. Those who are getting leaner are bouncing around between maintaining and getting leaner. The getting leaner, we can gather, live a highly active lifestyle and are the 1 percent best of us in fitness, health, and wellness.

They are our idols, models, heroes, mentors, actors, and musicians, and boy are they beautiful to lay eyes on. The 1 percent of getting leaners are our civilization's eye candy, the sought after, the immune.

Obliterating the unhealthy state of sedentary behavior and obesity are the primary objectives of obtaining your pandemic armor. You will never be healthy if you are fat. It is time to become active.

Do not fool yourself into believing otherwise. Do not let the assholes out there cajole you into believing body fat is okay, healthy, or the norm. Your survivability increases exponentially for every pound of fat you take off your carcass until there remains a minuscule amount left—just enough for the basic needs of the human body in the twenty-first century.

Bye-bye, body fat!

So long, sedentary me!

Adios, comorbidities!

And hello, maximal longevity and health!

So how do you do this? Let's start with obliterating sedentary behavior by replacing it with activity—and above all, stop getting fatter!

How do you stop getting fatter?

Easy! Eat less and move more.

The sum of this idea is EXERLEAN: EXERcise and be LEAN in all you do. I invented this portmanteau to clarify all that matters in the big scheme of physique transformation. There is only activity to burn calories and prevent calorie storage, eating lean, thinking lean, and existing in a lean body. This is the lasting scenario of health and longevity—the natural foundation for maximal immunity. Your pandemic armor.

First—stop being sedentary. Stop vegetating. Stop being a sloth. And start incorporating activity.

Activity is the opposite of sedentary. When you are moving, you are being active. When you are resisting, you have increased the intensity of your activity. Activity can range from mild and low threshold to high threshold and maximum intensity.

Threshold of activity refers to the level of burden or resistance placed on the musculature, skeletal, cardiovascular, and respiratory systems. Sedentary time has no resistance and therefore involves no activity threshold and low-challenge cognition. So, anything you do other than being in a still and restful state is taxing your body with whatever level of threshold you are burdening it with.

Seek physical burden. Maximize your threshold. Seek cognitive challenge.

The level of burden you place on your body will return a comparable level of benefit, including your heart rate, respiratory rate, resistance to muscles, and stress to the skeletal system. Minimum-threshold activity will result in low-level or minimal benefit to the body, medium threshold will result in moderate benefit, and high threshold, maximum benefit. The more activity you do, the more you will benefit, and the higher the intensity or burden, the higher the degree of benefit.

From the moment you wake up to the moment you go to sleep is your time for living life. Your awake time is your time to get shit done, take care of yourself, experience conscious thinking, and be fully attentive to your consequential actions. It is the only time of the day for you to make a difference, to produce, to love, to be a friend, to go to work, to experience meaningful and rewarding stuff, and to engage in your purpose. The awake day typically involves self-care, ADLs, IADLs, work, exercise, sex, recreation, eating, playing, and rest breaks when appropriate. The more you do, the more active you are, the more calories you burn. The higher the burden of activity on your body, the more calories you burn . . . and the benefits of exercise unfold.

Be careful with the rest breaks, though; they can kill productivity if overused and abused. I remind myself of this by telling myself, "I will have plenty of time to rest when I am dead, so until then, I will live." This is the premise of my drive to live my life fully engaged. *I do not have time for rest breaks.*

Rote exercise is the best activity you can incorporate to increase, maximize, and maintain your cardiovascular, respiratory, and metabolic performance. The data from over a century of evidence-based research, on the benefits of exercise, is monumental. There is no questioning the need for exercise. It is necessary for health and wellness. Exercise will change your life for the better.

The Benefits of Exercise

So, what constitutes as exercise? Have you ever exerted your body to the point you can feel your heartbeat—your blood pressure thumping the carotids in your neck, or pounding in your chest? Has your breathing been so labored, fast, and deep that you've had to pause, bend over, and put your hands on your knees to catch it? Have you ever sweated profusely during exertional activity? If you answered yes to any of these scenarios, then you have experienced the feeling and physiological results of exercise; you have endured the burden of resistance on the body.

You have done the work.

The heart, in particular your heart rate, is key when it comes to whether an activity or work counts as exercise. There are two main types of exercise in relation to what the heart and body do. The first type of exercise is *aerobic*, meaning "with oxygen." The body requires oxygen in the metabolic process of fueling the activity at hand; specifically, it consumes the oxygen. The second type of exercise is *anaerobic*, meaning "without oxygen." The body requires little or no oxygen in the metabolic pathway of fueling the activity at hand; in other words, it does not consume it. When it comes to changing your body, there are benefits to both aerobic and anaerobic exercise.

The 1970s initiated the mass trend of aerobics, specifically jogging, running, and machine exercise. The aerobic exercise trend has continued to dominate as the initial protocol of anyone who chooses to get in shape and lose weight. This is for good reason: it works. Aerobic exercise also improves cardiovascular health. But by choosing aerobic exercise over anything else, you may be neglecting the most beneficial form of exercise for losing weight and getting stronger—anaerobic exercise, otherwise known as weight training. We'll get to the benefits of weight training soon. First, let's go over the benefits of aerobic exercise.

Aerobic Exercise

If you want to get in shape, lose weight, or improve your health, then aerobics will benefit you. Aerobic activity must be a part of your plan for achieving your health and wellness goals. Aerobic exercise is anything you do that increases your heart rate, circulates your blood faster, and leads to labored breathing. If your heart rate is low during aerobic exercises, you are not doing aerobic exercise, are not going fast enough, or are in such high-performance condition (i.e., extreme athlete conditioning) that the exercise requires little effort. One way to know if the activity is providing aerobic benefit is to monitor your heart rate. For the most part, any heart rate under 100 is likely anaerobic. A general rule of thumb is that once your heart rate starts elevating above 100 beats per minute, aerobic exercise is beginning, and an even higher rate leads to higher benefit. A heart rate can be too high, though. Over 200 beats per minute is usually too high to sustain long term and should be avoided by most people. Max heart rate training is best left for athletes and those in extremely great physical conditioning. To figure out your *maximum target heart rate*, subtract your age from 220. So, if I am 45 years old, I would subtract 45 from 220, which is 175.

If you aren't an athlete in training, your *target heart rate* is your goal. To figure out your target heart rate for aerobic exercise, just subtract your age from 200. So, at 45 years old, I would subtract 45 from 200, which is 155. That means my target heart rate is 155 beats per minute. This method is not written in stone, it is just a guideline. I feel best at 138 to 148 beats per minute during long-duration aerobic cardiovascular exercise like using an elliptical trainer for forty-five minutes.

To figure out your overall heart rate range for aerobic exercise, subtract 20 or add 20 from your *target heart rate*. These are your low-end to high-end goals. At 45 years old, my aerobic heart rate range is 135 (155 minus 20) to 175 (155 plus 20) beats per minute. Any lower than 135 bears little aerobic benefit, and anything above 175 is overtraining for aerobic capacity, unless my goal activity thrives in this realm, as in the case of running a marathon or a short sprinting event.

So, any activity that is under your low-end target heart rate will be mostly anaerobic—without oxygen. The lower your heart rate, the less beneficial the aerobic exercise.

Aerobic exercise will help you build up your cardiovascular endurance for all endurance activities. Aerobic exercise has universal benefits on activity conditioning. Your level of conditioning refers to your endurance for whatever activity or exercise you are engaging in. For example, if you are highly conditioned for cross-country skiing, you will not necessarily be highly conditioned for a different activity like swimming. Aerobic exercise will benefit your potential for conditioning to any activity in general, but becoming highly conditioned at a specific activity requires repetition of that activity and a conditioning program specific to it. Therefore, conditioning yourself to a specific activity is usually best achieved through a combination of aerobic and anaerobic exercise.

Aerobic Conditioning

Becoming highly conditioned takes discipline, focus, and repetition. As I mentioned, becoming aerobically conditioned to an activity requires doing it over and over again. Time is the relative aspect to adjust depending on the level of conditioning you want to achieve. The more time you commit to an activity, the easier it will become for you to complete. Increase the time you actively engage in a specific activity, incrementally and progressively, and you'll increase the duration of your conditioning.

For example, say you want to run a marathon, but you don't normally run. Unless you condition yourself to finish it, you will fail. To build your marathon conditioning, first go outside and run. Run as long as you can at a steady pace until you cannot run anymore. When you stop, take your heart rate and write down how many minutes you were able to run before you had to stop. Then journal how you feel, what you ate before running, and how much post-exercise pain—*EXERPAIN*—you are in over the next few days. Then the next day, run again, but try running farther and longer. Again, run at a steady pace until you cannot run anymore, then record all data related to the run. Do this every day, over and over, until you finally can run the distance of a marathon or longer at a steady pace and without severe burden of stress. This is how you would garner marathon conditioning.

Pacing

When building up your conditioning, endurance, and power, you must pace yourself to prevent overtraining, early fatigue, and cardiorespiratory exhaustion. Pacing during an exertional activity places stress on the body. It is a combination of rest breaks and activity with the goal of incrementally increasing the length of time you can endure a stressful physical activity. For example, you can simultaneously build up your strength conditioning and activity tolerance so that you maximize your potential to run a full marathon.

Pacing yourself during an activity can also be done by adjusting your speed and intensity, with the goal of finding the "just-right" level of intensity to keep going until you're exhausted. Pacing yourself may also involve interval rest breaks as necessary, which allows your body to rapidly replenish itself so you can resume the activity.

I once rode a half-century bike ride with zero pretraining, fifty miles with only one ten-minute stop to eat and drink. I borrowed a bike and gel-padded shorts from a good friend whose passion is road biking. He and his wife once rode their bikes from the East Coast to the West Coast in one summer. He is the one who coaxed me into this half-century ride called Dam to Dam, a fundraiser for the Mike Utley Foundation, which went from the Rocky Reach Dam to Wells Dam and back. Mike Utley sustained a spinal cord injury on November 17, 1991, when playing as an offensive lineman for the Detroit Lions. I was Mike's trainer many years ago. He taught me many valuable lessons about life, performance, and becoming a champion. One saying that sticks with me is something a coach told him: "If you can do it, it ain't braggin'." This is true to the core. If you have done the work and developed an elite physical status or performance, it isn't bragging to say you can do it—it is fact that can be backed by execution without question. I was getting paid to be Mike's personal trainer, but I think I got much more out of the deal than he did. I ended up being an occupational therapist rather than a physical therapist because of something Mike said to me. The wise people you meet in life will usually give you a nudge in the right direction if you listen.

How was I able to complete this feat—a fifty-mile bike ride without training on a bike or building up my activity tolerance to cycling before the event? The answer is weight training. I am a knowledgeable personal trainer, a competitive bodybuilder, and a powerlifter. I know the key muscles specific to riding a bike, and I know how to train those muscles for strength, power, and endurance. So, that is what I did for a couple of months leading up to Dam to Dam. I focused on doing heavy squats for high reps—really high reps. Like, ten sets of ten for each exercise, at the maximum weight still allowing ten reps, yet at failure or near failure by the tenth. I finished squats with ten sets of ten calf exercises. Barbell squats is the best exercise a bike rider can do to maximize lower-extremity strength, power, and endurance. A combination of standing or seated toe presses finished off my calves. The second major exercise I focused on was barbell deadlifts. Deadlifts are a posterior-chain trainer (meaning they work the muscles on the backside of your body), especially for the glutes. The quads, glutes, and posterior chain are primary drivers in riding a bike. I knew that conditioning these muscles would prepare my body for an enduring bike ride—and it did. But barely—in the last couple of miles, my quads started spasming and cramping up. I could see my muscle striations quivering and losing control. I had to slow down to about twelve to fifteen miles per hour and coasted into the finish line, which was at Lincoln Rock State Park near Rocky Reach Dam. When I got off my bike, I nearly collapsed. After grabbing onto my friend, then a fence, I finally rested on a bench and let my quads chill out. I made it. I finished the job. Goal achieved—all because I paced myself and was able to condition appropriately.

Weight Training

Of all the activities you can do to develop and maximize your pandemic armor, weight training is the most beneficial. The benefits of weight training are compounding and exponential. Weight train one muscle, and the next day it is stronger. Weight train that muscle again, and it will grow stronger than it was after the previous workout. Habitual weight training is perpetually beneficial for your physical health, mental health, and overall ADL, IADL, work, and leisure functioning. Over time, you will increase your muscle mass, muscle strength, and metabolism.

The benefits of weight training far outweigh those of aerobic training or cardiovascular exercise. Weight training is the only activity that can force the body to add more muscle mass. More muscle means more metabolic potential—the ability to burn more calories at rest. The more muscle you have, the more calories you burn when you do nothing! Think about this for a second. This is the most valuable scenario in the fight against obesity and sarcopenia. For one, having more muscle mass is the opposite of sarcopenia, and having a higher metabolism at rest leaves you much less prone to gaining body fat. Wow! This is like getting royalty payments on a book you wrote. Muscle mass and the benefits of a higher resting metabolic rate that come with it give you future benefit—but unlike a book, muscles will shrink and wither away if you do not continue weight training. Use muscles or lose muscles.

Why is it that a very low percentage of people lift weights? Why has such a beneficial activity remained less accepted than sports, outdoor recreation, or rote cardiovascular exercise? There are three major reasons:

1. Worry about gaining too much muscle
2. Not knowing how to weight train, so not starting
3. Not seeing results fast enough

Let's address number one first: "I don't want to get too big."

Holy hell! Don't fall for this ruse—it's total bullshit. This is just an excuse to justify a person's reason for not resistance training. Ask any bodybuilder how easy it was for them to get their muscles, and they will laugh hysterically inside because they will see that you are clueless. If it were so easy to gain muscle and get "bigger," you would see a heck of a lot more muscular and athletic physiques roaming the world, wouldn't you? What we do see though is mostly overweight and obese people everywhere. Remember, 72 percent of us are overweight or obese! Even so, would you rather look overweight or athletic and muscular? It is unhealthy to be obese, overweight, or even anorexic and skinny-fat. It is healthy to be thin and athletic. Stick this in your brain forever—being too big or too muscular is impossible without taking steroids, insulin, human growth hormone, or all in combination. Even when these unnatural methods are involved, it will take a massive amount of work to "get too big." Plus, you risk your health and overall longevity. Being excessively huge from either obesity or muscle is unhealthy and unnatural. The most extreme of bodybuilders look superhuman and freakishly cool, but there will be a price to pay down the road for these individuals who sacrifice their health for their physique. The human body is not meant to be obese or freakishly superhuge in any capacity.

Don't let the media, tabloids, friend group lore, or jealous external influence deter you from improving your body. They will do this by instilling in you a message that weight training will make you get too big. The fact is that becoming obese is super easy, and getting muscular is super difficult. What routine weight training will do is decrease body fat, increase muscle mass, increase metabolic rate, maximize strength, increase overall power, improve on-demand stamina, and fortify the feeling of greatness while walking around in this well-prepared physique.

Some will argue that an obese person who lifts weights and does aerobic cardiovascular exercise is healthy. I've seen many doctors look at obese people from this perspective if vitals like blood pressure, heart rate, and cholesterol are all within normal limits. But those doctors fail to acknowledge the comorbid obesity. If a person is conditioned and strong because of regular training yet remains fat, it is because they continue to eat whatever the hell they want. Eating unhealthy causes a state of what I call *sweet blood*—hyperglycemia—and *sludge blood*—hypercholesterolemia, both disease-inducing states. (We'll discuss these crucial topics in a later chapter.) Of course, a fat person who lifts weights and exercises regularly is healthier than a fat person who is sedentary but doesn't fall for this falsehood of supposed healthiness. Body fat alone is the predisposing comorbidity for diabetes, heart disease, strokes, metabolic disorders, and a host of other badness. This is especially true in the aging population, who can no longer weight train and exercise due to obesity's toll on their joints and organs. The same goes for being a freakishly huge bodybuilder—at some point, the joints, tendons, organs, and supporting structures of the body, like the spine, will become overtaxed to the point of destruction. Nobody is immune from the effects of aging.

Let's address topic number two: "I don't know how to weight train."

Every weightlifter starts here. Nobody knows how to lift or feels comfortable lifting weights at the gym for the first time. Get over it—like every other first time at something, you just need to dive in. Initiation and execution lead to getting over the anxiety or fear of the unknown. You will develop your confidence one day at a time. The second day you go, you will be a little more comfortable and a bit more confident, until within a couple of months you are worrying more about whether you forgot your protein shaker or headphones.

If you have no clue how to use a piece of exercise equipment, then I recommend going to YouTube and searching "how to . . ." to learn the basics—for example, "how to weight train chest." There are millions of variations and techniques, so don't get anxious and spend too much time in this overview stage. After a thorough review of lifts and exercises, consider hiring a personal trainer. Most gyms offer a free orientation to the gym and will help you get started. This is a great opportunity for some expert input in the beginning. To keep that initial momentum going, pay a personal trainer until you get a firm grip on your workout. A personal trainer will not only guide you through a workout but also teach you how to exercise and train with weights, give you tips on how to diet, and ultimately teach you how to build your own workouts, eventually setting you free from needing a trainer. You will eventually become your own trainer, do your own research, and feel confident enough to try out new machines and lifts. This is the goal you should pursue. In time, you will be comfortable navigating the gym like a boss.

At one point in your life, you defecated all over yourself until you finally took the plunge and used the toilet for the first time. After that, using the toilet instead of a diaper became a whole lot easier, more fulfilling, and personally beneficial. The same goes for learning to lift weights and work out. At first, you are untrained, unconditioned, and weak—an incompetent weightlifter. With consistent weight training, you become proficient, conditioned, confident, and stronger. Now, why on earth would you want to go back to being incompetent? In time, all seasoned weightlifters become trainers, able to share their gymgoing knowledge with others. Trust me on this! When you become proficient in the gym, you will attract admirers and questions about your journey, positioning you to motivate others in their health journeys.

Now, let's review the third excuse: "I'm not seeing results fast enough."

A kindergartner cannot wish for college-level knowledge without learning and living it out first. In the movie *The Matrix*, Neo, played by Keanu Reeves, is able to learn kung fu by plugging into the Matrix, and after a few seconds of computer upload, he suddenly has all the knowledge of this complex martial art and just needs to execute the actions. The human brain cannot learn like this. There is no magic bullet for teaching a person kung fu or weightlifting. These are arts that requires skill. Only through learning, continued training, and time can a person master these skills and become proficient.

Not seeing results fast enough is the reality of life. The famous philosopher Parmenides stated, "Ex nihilo nihil fit," meaning "nothing comes from nothing." Remember what we reviewed earlier in this book about matter—you cannot get matter from no matter. Muscles and strength cannot be miraculously conjured with a snap of a finger, wishful thinking, positive vibes, or willpower. You can be grateful for your muscles and the strength, metabolism, and power that comes with them, but gratitude will not get them for you. Each muscle fiber must be created through the demands of weight training and built up with the building blocks of protein. The same goes for losing weight or body fat: it cannot magically disappear. You cannot burn more body fat than your activity level or calorie deficits permit. To gain muscle, you must place a physical demand on your muscles, at a high enough resistance to force your body to respond by building back with reinforcement. You can only burn off existing body fat by creating the nutritional environment to support thermogenesis (the process of burning calories to produce heat), entering a calorie deficit from your resting metabolic rate, and increasing your activity level to metabolize body fat for fuel. Both adding muscle fibers and burning off fat cells happen one fiber, one cell at a time. Author Darren Hardy refers to a gradual process like this as the "compound effect."

The compound effect is the buildup of seemingly insignificant, almost unnoticeable changes that added up over time, result in monumental and obvious results. Harnessing the discipline and power of the compound effect to achieve your greatness is what author Jeff Olson refers to as the "slight edge" in his book by the same name. The slight edge is similar in that great achievement—extraordinary results—comes from religiously *executing* tiny improvements, tiny disciplines, and seemingly insignificant accomplishments that through the compound effect lead to successfully achieving long-term goals. Your slight edge is your mindset, your beliefs, and your discipline to *execute*.

Long-term goals are the crucible of all great achievers, the ultra-rich, and the most influential people in history. Your dreams of a lean, muscular, strong, and aesthetic physique bolstered with maximum immunity, longevity, and high quality of life will result from maintaining your slight edge and compounding tiny, seemingly insignificant health-related positive thoughts and actions, until your long-term goal becomes your reality. This is the master key to all goal achievement, health or otherwise.

So, do not worry that you won't see results fast enough. Be patient and stay the course. Maintain your slight-edge mindset, and in time, the compound effect will lead you to achieving your long-term goals. Master this process, and you can do anything you set your mind to!

Indoor versus Outdoor Activity

There is something exceptional about outdoor activity. The primary benefit of outdoor activity is that it pulls you out of the house, out of the gym, and into the world around you. Fresh air cannot be overrated; something happens to the body and mind purely from being in the outdoors. Call it tranquility, call it the vastness of God—engaging in activity outdoors is a positivity booster, as well as a physical stimulator. Outside there are a plethora of physically challenging activities that can help you maximize your immunity, physical performance, and mindset.

Outdoor activities fall under aerobic or anaerobic exercise, depending on whether the activity is challenging enough to provoke your muscles, heart, and lungs to use oxygen or not. Trail walking, hiking, road biking, Rollerblading, kayaking, canoeing, downhill skiing, wakeboarding, mountain biking, cross-country skiing, snowshoeing, dirt biking, power sports—the list is long for what you can do outdoors that simultaneously engages the musculoskeletal and cardiorespiratory systems.

Instead of watching TV, playing video games, or doing nothing active, go outside. Do something mentally and physically stimulating outdoors. It is as simple as walking out your front door. Just keep walking, then walk faster. If you want more physical demand, head for elevated terrain. Breathe in the fresh air and allow your mind to be refreshed while putting your body through the physical activity it is begging for. Just like doing cardio on an elliptical or treadmill and simultaneously reading a book or listening to music, being outdoors alone will help the time go by faster. But for outdoor activity, it is not the music or book that occupies your mind, it's the trees, wildlife, architecture, colors, and smells that will mesmerize you. Like exercising on a treadmill, stationary bike, or elliptical for hours, you will reap the benefits of exercise—but take heed that when you're doing fun, mentally stimulating, and rewarding outdoor activities, you may just find yourself hours into it still going strong and yearning for more. Consider bringing a backpack with plenty of water, some jerky, fresh fruit, and a protein shake. Be prepared for changing weather, wear supporting footwear, and let someone know where you are going.

Know, though, that outdoor activities cannot replace the benefits of weight training. Weight training and bodybuilding prepares your body for anything in addition to weight training. I recommend combining outdoor activity with indoor aerobic and anaerobic exercise, with a primary foundational weight-training regime.

Here's an example of this scenario. John weight trains every muscle in a four-day split, Monday through Thursday after work at the gym. He does his cardio every morning Monday through Friday before work on an elliptical trainer while reading a self-help book. After work on Friday, he goes on an ATV or dirt bike ride on nearby trails. On Saturday, he enjoys hiking on a nearby mountain and taking pictures of the wildlife, and Sunday is a day of waterskiing on the lake. Your week could look similar to this or totally different. We all have different work, school, and home demands and responsibilities that we must work around to take care of our body, mind, and soul.

Hyperactive IADL and ADL

How you do everything matters. What do I mean by this? Remember, activity is the first and most important element of your pandemic armor because it helps you prevent the worst comorbidity—obesity. If you are obese, activity will help you reduce your weight. If you are not obese and don't ever want to be, activity will help prevent it. *How* you do everything is the foundation for your daily activity, and it can compound the benefits of your exercise.

Remember from chapter 7 that you should be hyperactive whenever appropriate. This includes IADL, the routine daily tasks that must be done, like housecleaning, laundry, and other indoor and outdoor chores. By turning your IADL into light exercise, not only will you will complete them quicker, leaving you with extra time on your hands, but you will also increase your calorie consumption, boost your metabolic rate, and burn off body fat.

The same is true with ADL. When I was young, my mother always advised my siblings and me to take "military showers," as she called them. A military shower referred to taking a shower quickly to save water and get the next person in (her mission to shower five kids daily in an assembly line). Taking a shower like this is an example of a hyperactive ADL. Other examples include getting dressed and any other activity you do to get ready for the day. An extra 30 calories burned in the morning may seem insignificant. But compound those 30 calories a day, and you'll burn off an extra 10,950 calories a year, which is 3.13 pounds of body fat burned or prevented. Not only that, but you'll gain at least thirty hours a year merely by being five minutes faster each day. When you look at it this way, the tiny gains from doing everything hyperactively lead to significant gains over time, whether in time, energy, or body composition. Hyperactive self-care,

ADL, and IADL take nothing other than a change in daily behavior and performance.

Balance is key. First do your physical work, which stresses your body, then rest your body to heal badass stronger and better. Eventually, you'll reach maximum immunity.

"R"
REST AND RECOVERY

A well-spent day brings happy sleep. —Leonardo da Vinci

Did you know that your body does its rejuvenation, memory consolidation, and remodeling while you rest? Sleep helps maintain your immune system, offers time for your body to replenish energy pathways, and maximizes your overall health and wellness. During work, the body is taxed like a business in commerce, left hollow of vital nutrient currencies and begging for replenishment. This is where a little rest and relaxation—a little R & R—becomes your ally in physical, mental, and spiritual transformation. A break in the day allows your body to remain in stillness. In this state of calmness, the damaged cells, the stressed tissues, and the depleted nutritional currencies of your body enter into replenishment mode.

In restoration mode, the body undergoes a miraculous process of replacing dead and damaged cells with new ones, reinforcing damaged tissues with higher-tensile strength and mass. The relentless search for the fountain of youth is right in front of your eyes—it is the human body. The human body is a miraculous entity of the self-healing, self-balancing, and autonomy needed to remain in the zone of homeostasis (physiologic baseline status). It's built with all the right stuff—*all parts included*—including the body's internal and natural fountain of youth. The fountain of youth per se is the natural physiological occurrence of healing.

There are no artificial means to reaching longevity, revitalization, or quick transformation that can beat your body's natural ability, so long as your body is set up to do so. Even if you score a prescription for HGH (human growth hormone), testosterone, or anabolic steroids, these artificial boosters are temporary and can come at a negative cost to both your wallet and your body. Through exercise, eating lean, and nutritional supplementation, you have the power to change your body. Through rest and recovery, your body does its magic. Only you have the choice to harness the power of your internal fountain of youth or live out the slow decay of your body and mind. You have to turn on the internal fountain of youth—the healing machine has a passcode, and without it, your immune system lies weakened, and you remain susceptible. Without healing, your body leaves the door open to hastened aging, sickness, disease, and disability.

Sleep

The first path to healing the body is sleep. Closing those heavy eyelids initiates a process that starts with the brain and moves to every cell in the body. During sleep, the brain removes toxins from the body twice as fast as that of nonsleeping hours. These are the same deadly toxins that are linked to Parkinson's disease, executive thinking dysfunction (your CEO), and dementia.

A full night's sleep improves cognitive functioning, which includes problem-solving, memory, and critical thinking. As the brain rethinks and dreams about events of the day, certain memories can be linked together, helping to connect the dots, you might call it, so you can solve complex problems. Amazingly, yes! You can derive solutions in your sleep, waking up with the answer to a problem. That's why sleep timed right can help increase learning potential by 40 percent—the improved memory retention and connection that in turn improves problem-solving when you access these memory banks later. Students need to sleep well to maximize memory retention and learn. So the night-owl student who is sleep deprived, especially if they also consumed alcohol or other drugs, retards their chances at maximum learning potential. Funny how being a college student and alcohol are synonymous when the opposite is the true path to learning and success. Hence why many billionaires are abstinent or strictly reserved to intaking any incapacitating substances.

Your emotional health may hinge on attaining quality, consistent sleep. During sleep, the brain recovers and replenishes neurotransmitters, hormones, and other chemicals that play a role in emotion, emotional lability, and emotional stability. This replenishment improves your emotional response to whatever stressors may come the next day.

Did you know that over 75 percent of Americans experience sleep deficits, dysfunction, or deprivation? This sleep deficiency is becoming epidemic, and its prevalence is rising exponentially. Experts predict that over 100 million Americans will be experiencing sleep problems by the mid-twenty-first century. Some research points to a rising global epidemic of sleep disorders affecting about 45 percent of the population as of 2022. About 30 percent of the world's population experiences some form of insomnia. Insomnia—the inability to sleep when you feel tired, want to sleep, or need to sleep—has also been associated with depression, other mental health disorders, type II diabetes, obesity, global cognitive dysfunction, and a plethora of other diseases. High sugar intake, caffeine, green tea, and smoking are also associated with increased insomnia.

Sleep or die. It is a necessity of life.

Active rest versus passive rest

Different forms of rest provoke the rejuvenation process. There is passive rest and active rest. Passive rest is sedentary time whereas active rest is in motion, yet at a level that allows simultaneous recovery. Unless you are at maximal intensity of activity, you are experiencing some degree of rest. What determines the difference between passive and active rest is the intensity of the activity and the time between peaks of intensity and rest.

When the body or the mind needs rest, you must not be active or mentally stimulated to reap the benefits of rest. Mental stimulation includes thinking actively and experiencing emotion. If your mind cannot rest when you lie still, it's counterproductive. The worn-out mind must unwind and replenish its nutrition, oxygen, hormones, and necessary chemicals for further work. The brain is constantly rewiring itself. New neurons form, and unused or unnecessary neurons are pruned back. This process uses resources. The body gets these resources through food, drink, and elements of the environment, like oxygen in the air and vitamin D synthesis triggered by the sun. The rejuvenation from rest outpaces the damage that has been done, so poor-quality rest or not enough rest won't heal or fully restore you. Maximal healing from high-quality, full rest leads to top physical performance and executive creative thinking skills.

How do you rest successfully? How can you make sure that your rest is of the highest quality and of adequate duration? You may not be able to control your sleep environment, the amount of noise in that environment, or other bothersome problems, but four parameters of rest are within your control. You can control your bed, the chemicals present in your bloodstream, the composition of your body, and time or the temporal atmosphere of your rest.

The Four Controllable Parameters of Rest

1. Your bed

The bed you make matters. Many of my patients report sleeping in a place other than a bed, such as on the couch or in a recliner. Of those patients who do sleep in a bed, many of them report having very uncomfortable beds. Most are adults over age forty. Now, I understand if a young adult cannot afford a high-quality bed or for the sake of convenience must be ready for the next move. But why, why in the universe would a mature adult still choose to sleep in a shitty, uncomfortable bed, on a frickin' cot, or on the couch? It is up to you to have a bed that fosters maximal-quality sleep.

According to a study published in 2009 by the National University of Health Sciences, the right bedding system can decrease back pain, improve quality of sleep, and reduce stress. Low-quality sleep is shown to lead to depression, anxiety, and increased stress. And stress in itself contributes to decreased quality of sleep or difficulty sleeping. High-quality, necessary sleep contributes to improved productivity, mood, self-confidence, and feelings of competence. Therefore, lack of sleep and poor-quality sleep must be prevented to capture the benefits of being well rested.

Research demonstrates that deficient quality and quantity of sleep are directly related to sleep surface. But the data are insufficient, or perhaps *too* sufficient, in determining what bed surface is best. Soft, medium-firm, and firm are all proven to be individually best for a multitude of benefits, including reduced back, neck, and shoulder pain, improved sleep quality, and comfort.

According to a four-week sleep study by B. H. Jacobson et al. to determine the best sleep surface, medium-firm bedding won the prize for reducing back pain by 48 percent and boosting sleep quality by 55 percent. This same study found that reducing overall pain and improving quality of sleep resulted in less overall stress. The study also noted that replacing an old bedding system with a new one improved sleep quality and reduced the negative side effects of an old or poor bedding setup. This study determined a bedding system to be old and outdated at 9.5 years. Given the amount of time the average person spends sleeping, a 9.5-year-old bedding system, at a rate of 8 hours of sleep a night, has received an average of 27,740 hours of use. That's 27,740 hours of body pressure, sweating, and friction tearing down the quality of your bed cumulatively over time. If you purchased a brand-spanking-new car and drove it nonstop for 8 hours every night at 25 mph, that equals 200 miles a day, 73,000 miles a year, and 693,500 total miles in 9.5 years. Most vehicles don't make it to 300,000 miles, let alone almost 700,000 continuous years. If a vehicle were used the same amount of time as a bed, the bed would far outlast the vehicle. Your bed takes on a huge toll.

Many studies have concluded that a person's stress tolerance is directly correlated to poor quality of sleep. Sleep deprivation has also been shown to increase the occurrence of anxiety and depression. In these studies, the positive results of changing to a new and improved bedding system are observed within the first week and sustained long term.

Most orthopedic surgeons recommend hard or firm bedding to reduce back pain. I have chronic back pain from decades of lifting patients and other patient care and have found that soft bedding surfaces foster my best-quality sleep. In particular, I like a twelve-inch medium-firm mattress with a three- or four-inch silky-soft memory foam topper. When I hit the bed, I want to sink into it and feel swaddled in plush comfort. This is my sleeping bliss.

Some research shows that body weight should be the crux for choosing a particular bedding type. I believe, however, that body composition and shape are the most crucial determinants. Take, for instance, a morbidly obese person. The morbidly obese come in a plethora of shapes, weights, and proportions, all out of the ordinary and dysfunctional. If the human body is contorted when lying in a bed, then discomfort, increased pain, and difficult breathing will result. This is why many, if not the majority of, morbidly obese people do not sleep in a normal bed. Most of my morbidly obese patients cannot sleep in a flat bed due to smothering in their body fat weight, so they sleep reclined or upright. At least half of my morbidly obese patients report sleeping in a recliner. However, to improve sleep quality and duration, obese and morbidly obese people must prioritize weight loss over bedding type, because bedding is engineered for the typical body shape. For the obese person, I recommend a power-adjustable bed so that the head of the bed can be raised to improve respiratory function and avoid symptoms of obstructive sleep apnea.

To ensure maximal-quality sleep, you can at a minimum avoid the worst of sleeping surfaces: the ground. Get an air bed, a cot, or a ground pad to avoid this. For daily sleeping, however, you should avoid these options and get a legit bed with a mattress and box springs or frame. Avoid purchasing a cheap, low-quality, poorly designed bedding system to save money. You are about to spend a third of your time in this thing. Choose the most comfortable and soothing bed type, brand, and adjustability based on your personal preferences, testing, research, and finances. There are many bedding stores, so try them all out if you need to. Your nighttime bliss awaits.

2. Chemicals in your bloodstream

What is running through your veins at night? The chemicals affecting your body are ingested through your diet as well as self-made by the body. Everything you eat causes varying levels of chemical reactions and processes in the body. The chemicals your body makes itself, in addition to the chemicals you ingest, are used in the biological effort to keep your body functioning and alive. For example, your body makes neurotransmitters, amino acids, hormones, cortisol, melatonin, and other chemicals that either promote or prevent high-quality sleep.

Neurotransmitters react with cells in the brain, including neurons, and the peripheral nerves the brain uses to communicate with every cell in the body. Serotonin is a neurotransmitter that's an important regulator of sleep and is heavily influenced by another chemical called tryptophan. According to research, tryptophan is necessary for the synthesis of serotonin. Serotonin is a precursor to melatonin, the primary chemical controlling sleep. So by depleting tryptophan, you suppress serotonin, which affects melatonin, therefore leading to poor sleep quality or sleep deficits. You can improve your sleep by eating foods high in tryptophan. You can handicap your sleep by consuming caffeine. Chemicals like these that are pulsing through your veins, especially as you approach your desired sleep time, can affect your mission to sleep well.

Functional foods. Nature supplies us with foods full of chemicals that help improve or impair sleep. Food engineers and scientists have created supplements and medicines, both over the counter and through prescription, that provide possible therapeutic benefits for sleep. Whether the consumable is provided by nature, engineered strictly by man, or comes from a combination of the two, it will be considered a functional food for the purposes of attaining high-quality sleep—and with it, maximal pandemic armor.

A chemical byproduct of energy consumption, physical exertion, and exercise is called adenosine. Adenosine in the brain acts as a central nervous system depressant; it maximizes your drive to sleep and suppresses wakefulness. Adenosine is also involved in regulating your sleep-wake cycles, including the light and dark of day and subsequent levels of melatonin. To ensure an adequate daily adenosine response, eat healthy, exercise, and do laborious work. Caffeine suppresses adenosine pathways, so you should avoid it completely if you want restful sleep.

Vitamins and mineral deficiencies, especially in zinc, vitamin C, vitamin D, vitamin B1, folate iron, phosphorus, magnesium, alpha-carotene, calcium, lycopene, and selenium, are associated with shorter sleep, difficulty falling asleep, and trouble staying sleep. Supplementing with these vitamins and minerals has been shown to improve subjective sleep quality, including the onset and duration of sleep.

Tryptophan supplementation has been found to improve sleep in middle-aged adults. In studies, consuming tryptophan-rich foods leads to less waking up during the night, improves the process of falling asleep, and increases sleep time, sleep efficiency, and restfulness. And vice versa—consuming tryptophan-rich foods early or midday negatively affects wakefulness, state of arousal, and mental acuity. Foods that are high in tryptophan include whole milk, salmon, tuna, turkey, eggs, spinach, oats, cheese, cherries, nuts, and seeds.

Melatonin is a natural chemical found in the body. Melatonin regulates our sleep and wake cycles. These cycles for most people revolve around light and dark periods of time. The light of the day suppresses melatonin production, which in turn heightens the intensity of wakefulness. When it gets dark, the body begins to produce melatonin, which in turn brings about the desire to sleep. For whatever reason, some people have low melatonin levels when it's time to sleep. Supplementing with melatonin can help improve sleepiness and sleep quality, as well as reduce insomnia. Melatonin supplementation can also counteract the negative sleep side effects of medications taken for high blood pressure, arrhythmias, and chemotherapy. Melatonin can also help people dealing with mental illnesses associated with insomnia, like depression, anxiety, and schizophrenia. The effects of jet lag can be lessened with melatonin supplementation, as can symptoms of migraine headaches and other pains. Melatonin is available over the counter.

Contrary to popular belief, alcohol does not promote sleep. Though alcohol seems to be a sedative and does help people feel relaxed, it has a negative impact on the ability to fall into a deep sleep and can interrupt sleep. Alcohol in moderation does not seem to negatively affect sleep as much as high alcohol consumption does.

Ghrelin and leptin are two hormones or natural chemicals in the body that regulate feelings of hunger and satiety. Ghrelin released into the bloodstream induces feelings of hunger and leads to a high desire to eat. Leptin, on the other hand, signals a feeling of satisfaction or feeling full, referred to as satiety. As stated in my book *EXERLEAN*, "ghrelin is the felon," which leads to hyperpalatable food addiction, overeating of these deviously engineered foods, and obesity. Go figure, sleep deprivation causes high levels of ghrelin and low levels of leptin. This out-of-whack hormonal imbalance leads to overeating. Sleep deprivation is also found to increase food-seeking behavior, especially of calorie-dense foods high in fat, salt, and sugar. Habitually overeating hyperpalatable foods over time leads to obesity and impaired sleep onset, quality, and duration.

In one study on female Japanese workers, high consumption of confections and noodles was associated with poor sleep quality, and a diet high in fish and vegetables was correlated to good-quality sleep. The study also found that missed breakfast and irregular eating patterns were associated with impaired sleep, as well as with frequent consumption of energy-promoting beverages and sugar-laden beverages. To promote high-quality sleep, avoid these drinks in the second half of your day.

3. Body composition

Being overweight is directly associated with snoring and sleep apnea. This pattern of disrupted breathing leads to impaired sleep. Generally, the body fat we think of is what we see: external. We see a chubby round face, a protruding stomach, larger buttocks, and smooth, marshmellowy body parts. What we fail to see is the excessive accumulation of fat inside the body. The fat inside you pads all your organs, including your tongue and mouth, your throat/vocal cords, your esophagus, and your lungs. In addition to the extra internal fat restricting your breathing system is the external pressure of a fat neck, potbelly, large buttocks, thick torso, and fat arms. All this pressure leads to impaired respiration, which manifests as snoring and obstructive sleep apnea.

There are non-obesity-related causes for snoring and sleep apnea, but these are much rarer and unpreventable. These causes can be enlarged adenoids, a deviated septum, an abnormal lower jaw, and enlarged tonsils, all of which may require surgery. These problems are also made much more serious when compounded with being overweight or obese. In most cases of obstructive sleep apnea, though, people are smothered by their own body during sleep.

Obesity-related hypoventilation syndrome (OHS) is a disabling sleep problem in which body fat compresses the victim's breathing system to the point of shallow breathing. Shallow breathing over time leads to carbon dioxide (CO_2) getting trapped in the lungs, in turn blocking fresh oxygen from entering. Over time, chronic CO_2 retention can lead to nighttime hypoxia and, in serious circumstances, daytime oxygen suffocation that increases the risk of major cardiovascular complications and death. A person with OSA needs to be under the care of their doctor and is highly likely to become dependent on using an expensive Trilogy home ventilator, a continuous positive airway pressure (CPAP) device, or a bilevel positive airway pressure (BiPAP) device, which delivers positive pressure while you breathe in and out.

If you suspect a sleep problem, talk to your doctor about it. You can get sleep studies that rule out or diagnose a disease and then start discussing treatment if necessary. My recommendation is to lose your fat until you have a lean, healthy body. At that point, I bet your breathing and sleeping impairments will be mostly if not fully resolved.

4. Time

Circadian rhythms take place in a twenty-four-hour cycle, or daily cycle. These are rhythms of physical, mental, and behavioral changes that are greatly affected by light and dark cycles. Your eyes sense light and dark and send signals to the brain, which in turn promotes a wakeful or restful state. Your metabolism slows at night and is dialed up during the day. Your body temperature lowers at night and rises during the day. You can develop good sleep hygiene by going to bed and waking up at the same time every day. This helps the body regulate itself and accommodate a regular routine of activity and rest. People who work the night shift are highly likely to experience chronic sleep deprivation and are at higher risk for obesity, mood changes, and cardiovascular disease. Working a nightshift career for the long term is directly correlated with a shortened life span. Lesser health outcomes are inevitable because it goes against the body's natural tendency to establish its circadian rhythms. There are ways you can lessen the negative effects of nightshift work, including going to bed and waking up at the same time on workdays and days off. Avoid high-sugar, high-glycemic, and calorie-dense meals in the few hours before sleep, and avoid high-fat meals in the second half of your day. And control your sleep environment as much as possible by making it dark and cool to simulate a nighttime scenario.

The best time to go to sleep is between 8:00 p.m. and 10:00 p.m., and the best time to wake is after 4:00 p.m. and before 6:00 a.m. According to the Sleep Foundation, healthy adults should get between seven and nine hours of sleep a night. For those over sixty-five years old, seven to eight hours of sleep will suffice.

Sleep affects your entire state of being. Chronic sleep deprivation and low-quality sleep lead to negative wellness and health consequences, like hypertension, decreased immunity, and poor disease resistance. Obesity, the number one cause for poor pandemic armor, is directly linked to inadequate and poor-quality sleep. Obesity is also directly linked to overeating and lack of physical activity, just as poor sleep is related to lack of physical activity (which exhausts the body), overabundance of unhealthy food consumption, and uncomfortable body composition. So, you have body composition, chemicals in the bloodstream, and activity versus rest all playing vital roles in the game of survival of the fittest.

Eat to live.

Sleep or die.

Fight or flight.

All in the name of survival.

To maximize the attribute of fittest in the chain of survival, you should harness the controllable power derived by maximizing your four parameters of rest.

Parameter #1: Get the highest-quality bedding system to maximize sleep quality and quantity. Do not watch TV here. Do not work here. Do not read here. Make your bed a place of rest and place of rest only.

Parameter #2: Control the chemicals in your bloodstream in the few hours before sleep. Avoid high blood sugar, high-glycemic foods, and high-fat and calorie-dense meals, and supplement with sleep-promoting chemicals like tryptophan, adenosine, and melatonin. Consult your doctor for other possible sleep aids like benzodiazepines, histamine, or other prescription meds. Avoid any stimulating chemicals in the eight hours before sleep, including caffeinated tea and coffee, other caffeinated beverages, stimulating herbs, alcohol, and smoking. Do not sabotage your sleep by ingesting non-sleep-promoting chemicals.

Parameter #3: Control the shape and size of your body. Do not smother your insides with excessive internal and external body fat. Go on a strict diet, start a weight-training cardiovascular exercise program, and change your body for the better. Build your muscles, strength, and with it, maximum immunity. Burn off your body fat and keep it off for the remainder of your life. Become the most athletic version of yourself so that you sleep like a war-torn and spent gladiator.

Parameter #4: Maintain healthy and regular circadian rhythms. Go to bed on time every day. Aim for seven to nine hours of good-quality, unbroken sleep every night. Wake up early to kickstart your metabolism, keep your circadian rhythms in sync, and maximize your calorie-burning potential. The sleep-timing protocol creates a daily routine that invariably develops into a profoundly rewarding, rest-friendly habit of sleeping . . . and sleeping well.

Modalities for Relaxation and Rest

The "R" in A.R.M.O.R. is all about how you prepare your body to repair muscles, joints, and organs damaged by your day of work, exercise, recreation, and relentless efforts, both physically and mentally. The "R" also stands for restoration, repair, and replenishment. Restoring your body's glycogen, ATP, and other energy pathways prepares your body for what is coming the next day. Replenishing the vital infrastructures bolsters maximal cognitive and physiological functioning. Your body and mind heal at rest and exhaust during work. To maximize your body's healing protocols, you can do more than get high-quality sleep; you can also focus on modalities that promote rest.

Modalities include activities, pastimes, or tools that help you heal faster, feel better quicker, and benefit therapeutically. Some of the most popular modalities are massage, acupuncture, yoga, tai chi, stretching, ice packs, heat blankets, contrast showers, cupping, electromuscular stimulation (e-stim) and transcutaneous electrical nerve stimulation (TENS), ultrasound, iontophoresis, traction, joint mobilization, laser and light therapy, prayer and meditation, kinesiology taping, cryotherapy, vibration, music, and hot tub therapy.

Ultrasound, iontophoresis, and taping are best completed under the guidance of a physical or occupational therapist. Acupuncture should also only be done by a specialist licensed in this modality. Cupping is a newer, less-researched modality and should not be administered or supervised without a certified professional. But most therapeutic modalities are safe enough to self-administer. Let's go over some of these easy-access modalities you can add to your arsenal of pandemic armor.

Superficial cold and heat

Superficial (meaning "surface") cold and heat are some of the most popular modalities because they are easy to implement and have instant therapeutic benefits. Superficial cold therapy includes a cold pack, a bag of frozen peas, or a cold shower. Superficial heat therapy includes a heat pad, a heated blanket, or a hot tub. Superficial heat, like a heat pack, can relax cramped or spasmed muscles, improve the range of motion in stiff joints, and minimize pain. Superficial cold, like using an ice pack on a painful knee, can reduce pain and inflammation, as well as shorten healing time.

Massage

Another popular modality is massage. There is nothing like meeting up with a good masseuse for a fabulous deep tissue massage. Many athletes use massage as a regular modality to shorten recovery so they can continue to bombard their bodies with weight training, exercise, and their sport of choice. Massage, especially deep massage, breaks up the buildup of lactic acid in overused muscles, which decreases pain, relieves muscle stiffness, and helps the muscles uptake the nutrients used in cellular healing. Massage can alleviate painful muscle cramping, spasticity, and spasms and help people relax, decrease stress, and enhance overall wellness. I have a Black Card membership at Planet Fitness because it gives me unlimited access to massage chairs and the Hydro-Massage beds and loungers. I complete at least one ten-minute session in a massage bed or lounger after every brutal bodybuilding workout to relieve my chronic mid-back pain and muscle spasms, as well as improve my circulation, range of motion, and state of relaxation. You might consider purchasing a massage chair for your own daily use to maximize your overall mental health and wellness.

Contrast shower

A contrast shower is bathing or showering in a hot environment and then moving directly to an ice bath or cold shower. This promotes better circulation, improved vascularization, and quicker healing and pain relief. My kids and I have our own fun way of taking a contrast shower. We get in the hot tub and get nice and warm, then jump out and make snow angels or roll in the snow for as long as we can endure, and then jump back in the hot tub. You can find your own way of doing this modality. It can be as simple as starting out with a hot shower, cleaning yourself, and then finishing by enduring the coldest water temperature for as long as possible. It is rare, but some therapy centers and gyms have ice baths and saunas for such therapy.

Stretching

Stretching has many therapeutic benefits. It can be done with or without equipment or received as a secondary benefit of exercises like yoga, tai chi, or other calisthenics that maximize joint range of motion. Maintaining maximal joint range of motion and flexibility can help prevent muscle strains, sprains, tears, and other physical stress-related injuries. As a person ages, it is important to stretch daily to keep joints and muscles limber and flexible, which in turn helps prevent injury and falls. Stretching also promotes circulation, joint mobilization, and pain reduction, which speed up healing.

When I was a teen and young adult, I did not need to stretch much. My stretching routine at the gym was about ten reps of an exercise without resistance, and that was it. Now that I'm a middle-aged adult, if I don't warm up and stretch before a strenuous workout or other physical activity, I feel the pain. As we age, our bodies stiffen. Figuratively, let's call this premortem or early rigor mortis (true rigor mortis is due to chemical changes on top of the old stiff body). In the aging years, muscle fibers atrophy, shorten, and lose their tensile strength. Joints lose lubrication, cartilage disintegrates, and tendons get thin. The closer we come to death, the stiffer our joints, muscles, and bodies become. You want to heed off death by staying flexible and mobile, so the older you get, the more vital it is for you to stretch daily and do range of motion exercises. It is totally possible for an elderly person to remain very flexible. I am talking extreme yoga flexibility. I have seen many patients over eighty years old who exercise daily, stretch daily, and continue to enjoy yoga posing. I recommend stretching daily and early in the day, if possible, to prepare your body for the upcoming stresses. Remember, the stiffer and more immobile your body gets, the closer you are getting to rigor mortis and death.

E-stim

The next modality I call shock treatment, but that may be unrepresentative and sound too undesirable. E-stim, or electrical stimulation, is an easy modality that is used on your muscles to help relieve spasms and cramps and improve circulation, which aids in healing. You can purchase an e-stim device in most retail stores, medical supply stores, pharmacies, and online retailers such as Amazon. The device comes with instructions, though you can also watch YouTube videos to see where to place the electrodes to maximally stimulate the target muscle or muscle group. Most devices are simply operated by placing two to four electrodes over the target muscle or muscle group, then controlling the intensity of electricity or muscular stimulation with an amplitude dial. Many e-stim units have preset programs that deliver predetermined electrical pulses to meet your individual goals, like therapeutic, deep tissue, or Swedish massage.

Light therapy

Light therapy has become popular for treating seasonal affective disorder (SAD). In the dark winter months to supplement the absent light of the sun, I receive my light therapy from going in a tanning bed for a short time when needed. Not saying tanning beds are healthy, but they do warm you up, provide bright-light treatment, enlighten your mood, and result in a healthier-appearing skin tone. There are much healthier, widely available ways for receiving the benefits of light therapy. You can add a light to your work desk, a mood lamp, a lighted salt block, light-boxes, dawn simulators, or specialty light bulbs. Sunlight itself provides vitamin D, kills bacteria and germs, gives you a tan that helps further protect you from sunburn, reduces symptoms of PMS, bolsters mood positivity, and improves sleep.

Red light (laser) therapy

Red light therapy, sometimes referred to as laser therapy, is a newer technology that stimulates the action potential of mitochondria, the little energy generators within our cells. This can result in higher energy levels, faster cellular repair, and overall better cellular health. Red light therapy is also used for improving skin conditions like wrinkles, scarring, and aging spots. Some research claims that red light therapy can promote hair growth, improve circulation, and decrease pain. Blue light therapy can help treat precancerous skin problems, acne, sunspots, and depression.

Visualization, meditation, and prayer

Amidst the chaos and calm of a day lies opportunities to daydream, to vacillate between vegetation and doing. In these cracks of time, you have the option to practice a purposeful method of thought designed for reaching your calm and directing your focus toward shit that matters . . . or linger in nothingness like a cauliflower. When you are bored, you are in turn boring, and when you cannot entertain yourself, you are led to wallow in your boredom like a cow to the water trough. You become stuck between something completed and nothing planned, the vacuum of which can suck you into the realm of unproductive wasted time. One of the most common suck holes of life is bingeing TV. The revolving escapade that we become enthralled in is more desirable than heroin to the addict. We become habituated to the paralyzing bombardment of sensory stimulation, the epic and twisted plots, the sex scenes, the porn, the immorality, the romance, the tears, and the near-blissful indolence that comes with it. The problem is the mental and emotional inability to engage in meaningful activities rather than succumb to the least-resistant path, all to fill the void of boredom, loneliness, and solitude. It doesn't end there, though. Once someone is drawn into the realm of television, they typically add in the excessities of hyperpalatable snacks and drinks, online shopping, YouTube, and social media. Basking in the kingdom of unproductive cadence leads to weight gain, sedentary time, and negative health, thus low immunity.

What can you do in the restful moments of the day to take advantage of boredom and make the time count for your betterment? The big three modalities are visualization, meditation, and prayer. These timekeepers have been used to reach higher ground since the dawn of Adam and Eve. Over eons, the methods have been modified to fulfill the needs of the time and person. Someone may use a method of purposeful thought for self-improvement, to find purpose, to achieve peace, to reach enlightenment, to center themselves, to talk with God, and so much more. You can fine-tune any method of purposeful thought to satisfy the immediate need of your psyche.

Visualization. Visualization is a tool to help you achieve success by reaching goals. It is a mental imagery exercise that can help you master an athletic sport, win a competition, give a speech or presentation, act in a theatrical production, topple an opponent, or win over the crowd in a job interview, to name a few. Many of the most famous, influential, and successful people in history use or have used visualization to reach their elite level of success. Carli Lloyd, a US Olympic gold medalist, banks her success on her ritualistic practice of visualization pre-performance. To prepare for the 2015 FIFA Women's World Cup final, she visualized the strategic proceedings necessary to score four goals during the game. Carli's four-goal plan did not fully materialize, but she did successfully achieve a hat trick, three goals back-to-back, in the first sixteen minutes of the final game. Visualization can also help you improve your sleep, lower your blood pressure, and decrease inflammation.

Visualization takes place in your mind, eyes open or closed, whatever works best for you. Imagine specifically the outcome, goal, or performance you desire. See yourself going step-by-step through the motions exactly how you want them to go. What do you see, feel, and smell? What is the temperature, the environment, the atmosphere, the weather? Make this vision as realistic as possible, and go through the process over and over again.

Research demonstrates that when you visualize things in this way, your brain and nerve system are activated as if you are engaging in the event itself. Imagining yourself executing the perfect long jump activates the same neural networks as the real event. The only thing missing is the muscle movement. This mental process helps you master the real process, deep-seat the motor plan, and condition the nervous system for maximal efficiency during the actual performance. This mental practice also helps spare your body and its muscles after physical practice, preventing physical exhaustion or fatigue when your body needs to rest. Bruce Lee is well known to have used visualization to master the martial arts. He would replay fight sequences in his mind until perfect execution was inevitable. He used visualization to clear his mind of limiting thoughts, striving to be formless, to "be like water," as he often said. Water forms to the shape of whatever container it's poured in and becomes the container. His vision to be formless like water during fighting competitions and while acting in martial arts movies gave all his physical maneuvers higher quality of flexibility, adaptability, and ultimately domination in his performance.

I have found visualization beneficial in preparing for the next day's agenda. Oftentimes before bed, I read over the materials and research I will use for my 3:00 a.m. writing jam. Then when I go to bed, usually between 7:00 p.m. and 8:00 p.m., I lie my head down on the pillow and imagine myself sitting in my writing chair, typing out words with ease and enjoying a productive writing session using the materials I just reviewed. This process helps my mind, body, and soul prepare for a successful session. Then, when my 3:00 a.m. alarm goes off, I am out of bed in seconds and writing within a few minutes.

Another arena where visualization has helped me and many other athletes is in preparing and memorizing upcoming bodybuilding posing routines. In a bodybuilding contest, a bodybuilding competitor has sixty to ninety seconds of onstage performance time to display their lean physique and symmetry by striking muscle-flexing poses and, in between each, a fluid movement transition. That's about ten to twenty different poses depending on how fast the transitions are and how long the body-builder holds the pose. The problem is that a bodybuilder's extremely restricted diet that's required to get lean enough to compete is mentally and physically taxing. In a restricted fat-burning regimen, the body-builder usually cuts or greatly minimizes carbohydrates, leaving them with sparing energy to get through the day—which includes all their other work, household, family, and exercise responsibilities—let alone practice a posing routine, which takes significant energy. So, due to energy deprivation, many bodybuilders like myself practice visualization to help them memorize and execute their routine onstage in front of hundreds of people.

Meditation. Meditation is another restful modality used to help a person find their center. Finding your center refers to establishing a connectedness to yourself and the universe around you. According to Healthline.com, there are twelve benefits of meditation: reducing stress, controlling anxiety, improving emotional health, enhancing self-awareness, lengthening attention span, reducing age-related memory loss, enhancing kindness, decreasing addiction, improving sleep, controlling pain, decreasing blood pressure, and being able to practice it almost anywhere. Research has shown that meditation improves your brain's efficiency in connectivity between the different regions of the brain, which helps you reap the benefits of meditation. There is also evidence that meditators have bigger brains than age-comparable non-meditators. Most experienced meditators will tell you that through routine practice, meditation can greatly improve one's mental and physical wellbeing and health.

According to Headspace, one of the most popular meditation apps, there are sixteen types of meditation, all derived from guided versus unguided and calming versus insightful meditation:

1. Focused attention
2. Body scan
3. Noting
4. Visualization
5. Loving kindness
6. Skillful compassion
7. Resting awareness
8. Reflection
9. Zen meditation
10. Mantra meditation
11. Transcendental meditation
12. Yoga meditation
13. Vipassana meditation
14. Chakra meditation

15. Qigong meditation
16. Sound bath meditation

What works well for one person might not work as well for another, so it is wise to try different types of meditation until you find the method that works best for you.

If you plan to meditate to improve your restfulness, find your center, or improve your overall health and wellness, there are many books available on the subject and many popular meditation apps like Headspace, Calm, and Aura. Audiobooks are my favorite method; hearing the material makes it go straight to my brain faster than visually reading it, which requires subsequent interpretation and organization by the brain. I have practiced Qigong, visualization, and tai chi forms of meditation, which have all provided benefits in different forms. Qigong, an ancient Chinese healing practice, is a gentle movement meditation requiring controlled breathing, a state of consciousness, and serenity to master one's energy. Visualization, as I mentioned before, mentally prepares me for writing and mastering my bodybuilding posing routine. Even though tai chi is not on the Headspace list, it nonetheless is considered by many as a form of meditation or "medication" in motion. This is similar to Qigong in the use of gentle and fluid motions, focused breathing, and finding serenity, but it also incorporates forms used to prepare for fighting, finding peace, and building a spiritual foundation. I have found it beneficial for improving flexibility, core strength, and balance.

Prayer. Prayer is likely the most ancient of all modalities. Prayer bridges the gap between us and God. It is the direct link to instantaneous communication with the one, the universe, the almighty. Prayer can be done from written sacred words, Bible scripture, or spontaneous and fluid expression of thought. According to the University of Minnesota's Taking Charge of Your Health & Wellbeing site, in an article titled "Prayer," there are six types of prayer: intercessory prayer, distant healing prayer, petition prayer, centering prayer, contemplative prayer, and meditation. Research demonstrates six main benefits of prayer, including benefits related to the mind-body-spirit connection, healing presence, relaxation, positive feelings, secondary control, and a placebo effect.

The power of prayer is both internal and intercessory or external. Meaning the power of prayer can be directed toward yourself or another person. When you pray for someone else, research demonstrates that your praying may help improve the other person's outcomes. For example, in a study completed in Seoul, South Korea, 219 infertile women treated with in vitro fertilization had over twice as high a pregnancy rate if they were prayed for compared to the women who were not prayed for. Another study on primates and wound healing demonstrated that after four weeks of being prayed for, the primates prayed for had better wound healing and improved blood markers than those that were not prayed for.

Conclusion

Sleep is the most important method for maximizing your rest and recovery. As you now know, your bed setup, your body composition, the chemicals running through your veins, and your sleep environment all determine the quality of your sleep. You must control these four parameters of rest to maximize the quality and duration of your sleep.

During the awake hours of the day, you will need to balance activity and rest. The low-intensity-activity hours allow for the benefits of passive rest and some intermittent replenishment and recovery. This is important because if you go balls to the wall in full-tilt work mode without rest breaks, your body and mind will go beyond the point of exhaustion, which leads to counterproductive chemical activity, fatigue, and delayed cognition.

Regardless of the pathway you follow to find your center and attain a restful state, you must aim to ultimately replenish and repair your body from all the damage, depletion, and exhaustion from its daily workload and stress. Rest prepares you for the next day of war. You see, a day of thinking, physical exertion, problem-solving, self-care, chores, driving, dependent care, running a business, sustaining an injury, and enduring mental and physical stress taxes your body, mind, and soul. You must get high-quality sleep to replenish your body.

Different modalities can help you rest so you can repair damaged body tissues, replenish your body, and heal. Use cold packs to treat inflammation or to relieve aching muscles and joints. Hot packs, electric blankets, and hot tubs loosen tight muscles and joints. Take a contrast bath to promote healing, improved circulation, and better health. You can try different forms of light therapy to see if they benefit you.

Prayer, visualization, and meditation are tools to help you de-stress and find peace and rest. The power of the mind, soul, and spirit can be harnessed through acts of visualization, meditation, and prayer. Try everything to find out what works best for giving you a little R & R.

In your quest to maximize your pandemic armor, you can now harness the power of "A" and "R." Let's move on to the next way you can minimize your susceptibility to disease and disability and maximize your immunity.

"M"

MODERATION

Happiness is a place between too little and too much. —Finnish proverb

You have likely heard the old saying "too much of a good thing." The idea is that something good in excess can become something negative. William Shakespeare is one of the earliest writers to use this phrase, which appears in *As You Like It*. In this play he writes, "Why then, can one desire too much of a good thing?" Our internal drive can make us go too far with anything good and not want to stop when necessary. That's when that good thing turns sour. Shakespeare's question can be answered with the simple truth that humans live with the results of everyday choices. We are highly sensory seeking, lean toward our comfort zones, and are often prisoners of our God-given power of free will. We have no accountability gauge. That's why we can easily overdo or underdo many things in life.

If you underdo a good thing like finishing a project, it may never get completed. If you overdo the sport of fishing, you will not have enough time for productive work. Listen to that new hip song you like over and over, and it will eventually lose its ability to stimulate you, possibly to the point that it turns sour to your ears.

An automobile or machine has gauges for the driver or controller to read in order to maintain a safe speed, monitor for overheating, or observe warning lights. The human body also should have come with gauges like warning lights so that we could easily monitor our bodies. That way, we would have accurate readings to make sure we would not run empty or become flooded, would not go too slow or too fast, would know when to say yes and when to say no. But the number of gauges the human body would need would be astronomical. Think about it for a second. We would need gauges for boredom, stress, play, sex (well, you can never have too much of that!), and so much more.

As a set of rules for survival, there are some choices that are not okay even in moderation. These deliver negative consequences that over time can lead to addiction, disease, disability, and death. One of our five worst symptoms of susceptibility, smoking, is on this list. There is no beneficial amount of smoking. It leads to black lung, cancer, COPD, emphysema, tracheostomies, heart attacks, and strokes, so it must be avoided at all costs. Another on the list of the five worst symptoms of susceptibility is illicit drugs. Methamphetamine, LSD, cocaine, angel dust, PCP, heroin, and others like them only harm the body, mind, and soul, leading to early and nasty death in most cases, let alone imprisonment and a cornucopia of other negative consequences. Things like this must be abstained from.

So, how do we know our limits? In our quest for maximum immunity, we must thin down the list of gauges to the most relevant. To do this, our goal must be moderation. *Moderate* according to *Merriam-Webster* means "avoiding extremes of behavior or expression: observing reasonable limits." Ah! *Observing reasonable limits*—sounds like we are talking *gauges* here. So, what gauges do we need to home in on to help us develop our pandemic armor and reach maximum immunity?

A Gauge for Food

The most important gauge must be for food consumption because the worst possible symptom of susceptibility is excess body fat. Moderation of what you eat maintains the status quo. If a person is lean and has a healthy body weight, then moderation is the key to food intake balance. Moderation of food intake will prevent a healthy-weight person from getting fatter. On the other hand, a skinny, malnourished person may need more than would be considered moderate food intake until they reach a healthy body weight and nourished body, at which point they can practice moderation. However, moderation will not help the obese person lose weight. Excessive food consumption leads to obesity. If an obese person transitions from excessive food intake to moderate food intake, then maintaining that state of obesity will continue. Therefore, moderation with food does not work for fat people because it is too late to be moderate. Restriction is needed for them to lose weight.

When it comes to food types and quantities, moderation is subjective. How many cookies are too many or not enough? How many vegetables are too many or not enough? For the overweight person, there is no safe quantity of donuts, cookies, or candy. These hyperpalatable foods will only make an overweight person fatter. Remember the first rule to building your pandemic armor and maximum immunity comes from the "A" for activity: to stop getting fatter.

If you are overweight, obese, or morbidly obese, then you cannot follow the same moderation rules that a lean, healthy person follows. If you are lean and healthy, you can safely assume that if you want a cookie or candy once in a while, you will likely not store it as body fat but metabolize the energy from it for work, exercise, and recreation. So long as you are lean, active, and healthy, keep doing what you are doing because it is working. But for the fat person, stop eating that shit! Excess body fat needs to be metabolized, and if you're eating hyperpalatable foods or too much food in general, then you will not burn off any body fat. In fact, you will most likely be getting fatter. If you are overweight, restricting calories, carbohydrates, and fats needs to be the focus until you're walking around with a lean and healthy physique.

A gauge for calories

The food gauge can simply be a calorie measurement. If you are overweight, your food gauge needs to lean toward low calorie. If you are frail and malnourished, then you likely need to increase calories to maintain lean body mass, avoid sarcopenia, and ensure you have enough energy for activities and work.

A gauge for carbohydrates

If you are an extreme endurance athlete with a lean body, then you will need a gauge for not only calorie intake but also carbohydrates. A gauge for carbohydrates is a sugar or energy gauge. Endurance activities and strenuous work benefit from higher-carbohydrate intake to ensure adequate energy for work and replenishing muscle glycogen (fuel for energy stored in the muscle). If you are fat, then the carbohydrate gauge requires low-carbohydrate intake to restrict your energy consumption, in turn forcing your body to use its fat for energy.

A gauge for protein

There are many kinds of protein, ranging from plant to animal to supplement. All protein sources are not equally beneficial to the human body. Protein kinds are scored on a scale called the biological value (BV) of protein. The higher the biological value of the protein source, the higher benefit the protein source is for the human body. Protein is the most important food gauge for maximum immunity, health, and wellness. Lean body mass requires protein to repair, replenish, and construct new muscle tissue. At a minimum, we must consume enough high-quality, high BV protein on a daily basis to preserve lean body mass and prevent sarcopenia. Remember, sarcopenia is one of the top five symptoms of susceptibility. In addition, your immune system itself hinges on how much lean body mass you have. Studies show that a higher presence of muscle mass leads to higher immunity. White blood cells fight infection, and the more muscle you have, the more white blood cells you have, thus increasing your infection-fighting potential.

For the fat or lean person, lean high biological value protein intake cannot fail. If you are fat, replace carbohydrates and fats with lean high biological value proteins. Doing this will automatically lower your energy consumption and turn your body into a body fat incinerator while making sure you do not burn lean body mass for energy. Protein intake preserves lean body mass in a low-calorie, low-energy, and thermogenic environment. If you are lean and healthy, strive for adequate lean high biological value protein consumption to build more muscle and increase your immunity potential.

A gauge for fat

Fat is minimally necessary for health. This calorie-dense, high-energy food should be monitored and restricted at all times for both overweight and lean people. Too much fat long-term turns the body into a heart-attack and stroke-prone machine. Eating excess fat is a guaranteed way to accumulate body fat and eventually become obesity. Considering that there is fat in almost everything you eat, there is no need to worry about consuming enough fat, in the case of digestion and assimilation of fat-soluble vitamins. To ensure that you capture the benefits of omega fatty acids, take a good-quality fish pill daily. I use the Kirkland Signature Wild Alaskan Fish Oil 1400 mg softgels from Costco, which offers omega 3, 5, 6, 7, 9, and 10 fatty acids. Omega fatty acids are shown to decrease inflammation, improve cardiovascular health, promote healthy skin and hair, help regulate blood sugar, and play a critical role in immunity. Also, during the week, I will eat a minimal number of nuts, as they provide omegas, and I cook all foods in a little olive or canola oil, which are considered healthy oils.

A Gauge for Sleep

Don't sleep your life away. There is a time for rest, play, and work. Balancing each is paramount to maximum health and immunity. Too much sleep is unhealthy. The body needs to metabolize and engage in self-care, ADL, and work, which cannot be done when you are sleeping. All the while, you must maintain the "R" in A.R.M.O.R.: rest + relaxation + recovery.

As we talked about earlier, research shows that seven to nine hours of high-quality sleep is all we need. If you sleep six hours a day, that leaves you with the benefit of eighteen hours of awake time to be productive. However, getting six hours of sleep might eventually lead to sleep deprivation, which can be unhealthy overall and lead to fatigue, thus lowering quality productivity. If this is the case, then you may need to get a few days of extra sleep to replenish your body chemicals, hormones, and stored energy. Get twelve hours of sleep a day, and you will leave yourself with only twelve hours of productive time. If you sleep twelve hours and work an eight-hour shift with time to get ready and commute, then you have less time for work, exercise, or play. Oversleeping like this also leaves only twelve hours of the day to eat and metabolize everything you eat compared to a person who sleeps only seven hours a day. So, if a person needs 2,000 calories a day, the seven-hours-of-sleep person can metabolize 118 calories an hour during awake hours compared to the twelve-hours-of-sleep person, who has to metabolize 167 calories an hour during awake hours. The twelve-hours-of-sleep person therefore has a higher probability of storing excess calories as body fat purely based on having fewer active hours of the day.

More and more evidence is coming out on seven hours being a moderate or premium amount of sleep. The lowest morbidity and mortality rates are associated with getting seven hours of sleep. Research demonstrates that habitual oversleeping is associated with many diseases and causes of death, including diabetes, heart disease, stroke, increased pain, cognitive deficits, obesity, decreased fertility, depression, and inflammation. Stick to your sleep gauge of seven to nine hours.

A Gauge for Work

We can all relate to too much work. It is rare to hear someone complain about not having enough work. But in reality, not enough work is exactly where most people are. It is human nature to follow the path of least resistance, and work is resistance. So, most of us strive to work as little as possible to survive and support ourselves and our families. But some people seek out more work, more money, and more power. They are hell-bent on fighting against resistance and have likely mastered balance in all elements of life. They are in a flow state more often than most other people.

The consequences of not enough work are obvious. Not enough work leads to poverty, debt, low socioeconomic output, and financial stress. Not enough active work leads to obesity, sarcopenia, and deconditioning. So how much work is too much on the gauge of work?

According to the World Health Organization (WHO), overworking is fifty-five or more hours per week. Research shows that working fifty-five or more hours a week compared to working thirty-five to forty hours a week leads to a higher risk of disease, disability, and death.

How much work do we need to eliminate the negative side effects of no work at all? One mega study, a meta-analysis, found that a male needs to work only one eight-hour day a week to prevent the negative consequences of no work at all. The same study shows that a female needs at least twenty hours of work a week to eliminate the negative effects caused by no work at all. One guarantee, man or woman, is that no work equals broke-ass poor and susceptibility to deconditioning, muscle atrophy, and obesity.

Based on the evidence, I recommend working as much as you can while maintaining your emotional health, mental sanity, and spiritual enlightenment and balancing your energy expenditure with energy renewal. This is the key. The more you work, the more money you make. The less you work, the less you make. This is true no matter how much you make per hour. The more active and physically exerting your job is, the more likely you are to be lean and healthy. But if you are overworking, you will live with the effects of overtraining, exhaustion, and possibly chronic fatigue. According to the research, you must work between eight and fifty-five hours a week to capture the maximal benefits of work and prevent the negative effects of overwork.

If you work a thirty-two- to forty-hour workweek as most working Americans do, then think about how many days a week you work versus how much time off you have. For example, work four days a week, and you automatically get fifty-two more days off a year than someone who works five days a week. You may have to work more hours in a day working four days a week, but the juice is worth the squeeze when we're talking about gaining fifty-two days off. This does not include paid time off (PTO), vacation pay, or paid sick days. So, add your annual PTO to your extra fifty-two days off a year. Wow! What a difference this will make in your personal life. Short-term sacrifice for long-term reward.

Work five days a week, work 260 days a year minus PTO.

Work four days a week, work 208 days a year minus PTO.

Of course, if you work three days a week, you get even more time off plus PTO. Tragically, if you work six days a week, you ultimately work 312 days a year minus PTO. Many jobs do not include PTO, so the more days a week you work, the less personal life you have.

In the mission to achieve moderation in the amount of work you do, you must look at the key parameters of work:

1. *The monetary value of work*, meaning the more you work, the more you make. If you need more money, you need to work more hours a week. If you are already working maximum hours a week, then the only way to increase your income is to get a promotion or move to a higher-paying job. With either option, you must be worth the investment for the employer. This typically means you need to gain higher education, specialize, or improve your skill set. No one deserves to get paid more than what they are worth based on output, specialization, and skill set.

2. *The negative effects of no work on health and wellness.* Do not work less than one day per week and no more than fifty-five hours a week to maintain the maximal health benefits of work.

3. *The time value of work versus no work.* Balance days of work with days of no work to find your happy place. Simple time management can improve your outlook on work and lead to working less and having more time off. Strive to work the least number of days possible, yet continue to earn the income

necessary to maintain the lifestyle you desire. You will simultaneously maximize days off for mental, emotional, spiritual, and physical energy restoration.

A Gauge for Stress

Stress comes in different forms. Physical stress stimulates muscles, bone, and connective tissue density and growth. Sedentary stress is the overabundance of stored energy in muscles, the bloodstream, the gut, and body fat. Mental stress is an imbalance in life enjoyment versus disenjoyment, which leads to high blood pressure, increased body aches, chronic fatigue, and possible psychiatric issues. Sleep deprivation leads to emotional, mental, and physical stress. Stress from pain is common as we age. Middle-aged, aging, and elderly populations deal with different forms of chronic nagging pain, usually from work involving repetitive lifting, exertion, and other cumulative microtraumatic injuries. Emotional stress hits us when personal, social, or relationship turmoil or trauma has occurred. Cognitive stress varies depending on the intensity of your daily critical thinking, problem-solving, and memory retention. No long-term cognitive stress leads to brain deterioration and dementia, cognitive slowing, poor judgment, early disability, and death. Just like a muscle needs physical stress to stay alive, the brain needs cognitive exercises and strain to stimulate continued capacity and function.

Regardless of its origin, stress must be strategically managed. There are benefits of stress and harmful consequences of stress. What kind of stress you are taxed with matters. If you have plateaued or are failing to progress, you need more stress. You need to put yourself back into the game, as a coach would say. Stress must be near the breaking point—to the point of failure—to stimulate growth and repair of lean muscle mass, increase metabolism, break mental barriers, awaken the spirituality inside, and intermittently jolt the mind, body, and spirit out of indolent and unstimulating comfort zones. On the contrary, no stress can't lead to maximum success, physical health, and immunity. No stress at all leads to muscle atrophy, bone decay, and weakness; leads the mind to wander and then halt; and leads your overall being to become indolent, boring, and unproductive. A life absent of pain is a happy life according to Greek philosopher Epicurus, but without pain, there would be no pleasure. Without pain, what sign would indicate that you pushed the envelope hard enough, that you struggled or gave it you're all? Pain is a sign of the laborer, the hero, and the conqueror. But pain can also be disabling. Excessive pain is a sign of overstress and mistakes. Disabling pain needs to be undone with relaxation, rest, recovery modalities, and possibly medical oversight or medicine.

Seek stress.

Seek pain . . . but not too much. There is beneficial pain and non-beneficial pain. Delayed onset muscle soreness is good pain—temporary pain from engaging in a hard day of manual labor or a great weight training session. No pain, no gain! the coach would say. I say no strain, no pain! However, injury or traumatic pain is bad pain. The body needs just enough stress to stimulate muscle growth, strengthening, and repair—and delayed onset muscle soreness or pain will exist afterward if the stress on the body was executed correctly. Just enough stress and pain also trigger higher bone density and more joint stability. The mind, body, and soul need stress and pain as signals for change—you are either not pushing hard enough or pushing too hard. How much stress? How much pain? Just enough to keep your mind sharp. Just enough to keep you feeling something, and just enough to keep you attentive and alive. When in doubt, push or try harder. Increase the stress, workload, and effort to the brink—then back off the intensity or duration when needed. If you are new to exercise training, athletics, or manual labor, I recommend you seek a trainer, a mentor, or a coach to help you learn how to strategically stress and manage pain in your body.

The trick with moderation is to find your positive place, to balance the elements of emotional, cognitive, physical, spiritual, and sedentary stress and pain. Everybody works differently—mentally, emotionally, and physically—and what may be too emotionally stressful for one person might have zero effect on another. For the physical part of you, you need to exercise, lift weight, and remain as hyperactive as possible to get stronger, remain strong, and prevent muscle wasting and obesity. The emotional side of you needs to feel. Seek feelings of reward, pleasure, and discomfort. The discomfort is caused by exercise, being social, and maintaining good relationships. This is where sedentary stress needs to be managed. If you are too comfortable and too lazy, then your body will retaliate with lower immunity and eventually sickness, disease, and poor quality of life. The spiritual side of you can lift you out of a rut, drive you to seek renewal and reward, and motivate you to break out of your comfort zones. In the end, would you rather become a cognitively disabled and demented retiree or remain cognitively intact, able to make decisions for yourself and recognize your loved ones? You chose your fate. Your body and brain need exercise. They need to push against resistance more than not. Fight indolence and thought wandering. Whether it's weights or a difficult crossword puzzle, do something hard as much as possible. Strive for success to the point of discomfort and pain. Then and only then, you will know you are alive. How can you know what moderate is if you don't push to the point of failure, discomfort, and pain? With a taste of it, you will know when to back off to the point of moderation. This is when the body, mind, and soul thrive, and from these results come maximum immunity.

"O"
OBLITERATION

Sometimes only pain can obliterate pain. —Alma Katsu

Art is the elimination of the unnecessary. —Pablo Picasso

Obliterate everything from your body that is unnecessary and possibly causing pain.

It is the unnecessary elements of a man that develop into low immunity, sickness, and pain. Obliterating the seeds of sickness becomes the absolute derivative to donning pandemic armor and experiencing maximum immunity. —John Blade

Obliterate Body Fat

There is no need to have body fat. Body fat is a sign of overconsumption, overeating, and lack of exercise. Body fat is a symptom of a disease, which hampers immunity. The overwhelming majority of people becoming gravely ill and dying from COVID-19 have been fat and deconditioned. COVID-19 loves body fat! Based on frontline observations, body fat must be some kind of fuel for COVID-19, its number 1 leverage against humans. The more of it you have, the more leverage it gives COVID-19 and other pathogens to fuck you up. So, you must get rid of body fat.

To obliterate your body fat, you will need to do uncomfortable and unfamiliar acts. You will need to feel the pain of real transformation. How can morphing an obese body into a lean and mean machine feel pleasurable? It can't. The opposite of pain is pleasure, and it took years of excessive pleasure to earn your overweight, fat, or obese physique. Therefore, pain and discomfort are the remedies for treating body fat. Specifically, the mental and physical pain and discomfort from fasting, restricting calories, and eliminating hyperpalatable foods.

Just like the heroin addict must detox and feel the discomfort and pain of withdrawal, so must the food addict who loves hyperpalatable foods. These tasty engineered foods are a massive contributing factor to obesity, triggering the same areas of the brain as heroin, crack, cocaine, and methamphetamines.

Abstinence is crucial. Detoxification and withdrawal are inevitable. This is the true path to obliterating a bad habit. And seeding a new healthy habit requires daily focus, care, and nurturing for it to take root. It takes discipline, patience, and time to make what was once comfortable uncomfortable, and what is at first uncomfortable comfortable. Food restriction and fasting are physically, emotionally, and mentally difficult. It is very uncomfortable to restrict something that your brain, the cells of your body, and your mind are habitualized or addicted to. What determines your present habits form out of daily rituals. That's why physical transformation and weight loss is a climb into the fires of hell. With discipline you push, restrict, and improve. As you're dancing in the hell of hunger cravings that an empty-bellied zombie cannot fathom, you must have impulse control. You must fend off temptation and the glimmer of hyperpalatable foods that try to seduce you, and have self-confidence to heed off the naysayers, a-holes, and loved ones who will be offering you the foods you cannot have . . .

the donuts of hell. You must persist. After a couple of weeks, as your bad habits and addiction dissipate, you will climb out of the bowels of hell and into the enlightened realm of physical health, mastering control over what you eat and don't eat. Your motivation will build as you observe your body becoming leaner and leaner every day. The diet grind will become easier and more comfortable with continued practice. You can win the body of your dreams. Anyone can. You just have to do what is necessary to transform your body. The first step to controlling weight gain and creating an environment of total body fat incineration within your body is to control your blood.

Obliterate Sweet Blood

The sum of obesity is derived from the combined attributes of indolent behavior, sedentary time, the absence of work, an overabundance of energy, change avoidance, insulin, and sweet blood. Of all the different attributes that lead to obesity, the ultimate primary sin, the primary cause, for body fat weight gain is sweet blood.

Sweet blood is blood that is saturated with glucose after you eat carbohydrates. Carbohydrates are broken down by the digestive system and converted to glucose, a sugar that is pumped into your bloodstream. Glucose is pure energy that's used in cellular metabolism, as fuel for the brain and other organs, and as the primary power supply for work and exercise. Glucose is sweet because it is pure sugar. Put this shit in a wine glass and drink up, because you won't know the difference between sweet blood and dessert wine.

This sweet blood running through a carbohydrate consumer's veins and arteries triggers insulin release. Insulin is the body's most *anabolic* chemical (i.e., a chemical state promoting repair of damaged tissues and growth of new muscle fibers) that tells the body to use calories—right frickin' now! The faster calories are assimilated and processed by the body, the more excess calories are stored as body fat rather than used for energy. The more insulin that is released, the faster calories will assimilate. The faster calories are delivered to the body, the less of a chance you have to burn them off as fuel for work or brain power, and the greater the chance of storing them.

God holds us accountable for our actions; otherwise, God would have designed the human body to poop out all excess calories rather than store them as body fat. It would be much healthier and more functional if the human body did not have the capacity to store extra body fat. The human race would remain 100 percent lean, beautifully shaped, and geared toward maximal function. Ha! This is not how it is, though. The power of free will and the consequences that come from gluttony, indolence, and addiction are real and remain a constant strife.

We all dance with the devil at some level or another. Sweet blood is the devil, which sends out its minion, insulin, which in turn rewards us with layers of disabling body fat, metabolic disorder, and disease. The reward, in reality, is the punishment of being gluttonous. All actions and decisions have either a benefit or a cost. The debt of sweet blood must be canceled out with action, activity, manual labor, exercise, or recreation.

I told you that insulin is the most anabolic hormone in the human body. Anabolism is to growth as warmth is to the sun. It is an environment within the body needed for you to get bigger, better, and stronger. Anabolism is a good thing for an anorexic, a sarcopenic, a postchemotherapy patient with muscle atrophy, an athlete, a manual laborer, a hunter/warrior, and for sure those who strive to build their bodies better. Some extreme bodybuilders inject insulin after eating a calorie-laden meal loaded with protein and nutrients so that their body will assimilate the nutrients rapidly, thus creating a growth environment that helps them get bigger. Do not do this! This is dangerous. You could accidentally kill yourself messing around with pharmacologics, insulin, and blood sugars. Only insulin-dependent diabetics should be using injectable insulin as their bodies do not produce or manage it correctly, and this should be under the guidance of their primary care doctor.

All foods trigger a release of insulin. What matters in the big picture of body weight and metabolism of body fat is carbohydrates. To manage your blood sugar, or sweet blood from insulin, you must focus on carbohydrates. Carbohydrates are the dominant determinant of the release of insulin, both its quantity and duration. Meats, dairy, fish, and eggs are great high biological value protein sources that influence insulin but minimally affect blood sugar. These foods are different from carbohydrates in that they are bulkier, take longer for the digestive system to break down and assimilate, and are highly valued by the body for cellular repair, new growth, and immunity. Your chances of getting fat eating lean, high-biological value meats, dairy, fish, eggs, and similar protein sources is null. Focus on managing your blood sugar, obliterating sweet blood, and monitoring carbohydrates using the glycemic index (more on this process shortly).

Remember this as though your life depends on it: *Your body will not metabolize body fat in a hyperglycemic state.* In other words, if your blood is sweet, your body cannot burn off body fat. The body must metabolize all that blood glucose before it can turn to body fat stores. Therefore, the end game of obesity is to ultimately prevent sweet blood from running through your veins. In instances of extreme athleticism, the athlete can aerobically burn off glucose, glycogen, and body fat stores simultaneously, but this is an unrealistic goal for the average human, especially a deconditioned fat one.

Carbohydrates come in different types, and each type triggers a different intensity of insulin release and a different response by the body to compensate for it. There are slow carbs (aka low-glycemic carbs), moderate carbs (moderate-glycemic carbs), and fast carbs (high-glycemic carbs). Slow, moderate, and fast refer to the speed of digestion and glucose delivery into the bloodstream, and the subsequent insulin spike based on the type and quantity of carbohydrate you've consumed. You eat carbs, and your blood sugar is directly affected.

So, is sweet blood the devil, or are carbohydrates, which create sweet blood and the corresponding weight gain? Something to think about.

The second a carbohydrate is identified by the brain, the digestive process is initiated. The brain is first enacted by the aroma, which then signals the stomach to get ready, to get the epigastric juices flowing for digestion. Your salivary glands secrete saliva to moisten your oral cavity to prepare it for tasting and chewing. As you taste the food and grind it up, your blood is already priming for insulin release, if not already spitting out a little into the bloodstream to manage the fast sugars in your saliva or those you've swallowed.

Think about this? When you approach a Kentucky Fried Chicken meal, what is the first thing that happens? When the aroma of that secret seasoned battered and fried chicken, coleslaw, and buttery honeyed biscuits hits your olfactory bulbs, it instantly triggers the hunger and desire areas of your brain: "Must eat. So hungry." The signals your brain delivers are intense because these hyperpalatable foods are scientifically engineered to do just that—to trigger the same areas of your brain that heroin, cocaine, and speed trigger. You lose control. You may not even be hungry. But you will stop and enjoy the blissful tastes, smells, and satisfaction of that KFC meal. Listen to me—it is not worth it! Not if you are overweight or obese. The cost of consuming calorie-dense, hyperpalatable foods is continuing your perpetual unhealthy, immuno-compromised overweight or obese state. If you have a lean and mean body, KFC is okay in moderation. Otherwise, no. You can't have any. Not until you get lean, strong, and immune.

If you can prevent or at least minimize sweet blood and insulin, you can minimize weight gain. To minimize insulin, you need to minimize and ultimately prevent sweet blood. To prevent sweet blood, you first need to obliterate hyperglycemic carbs, or fast carbs. This includes foods like cookies, cakes, donuts, pies, candies, energy bars, syrups, jellies, jams, sodas, and some fruits. If it is sweet, it is most likely not conducive to weight loss as it will likely sweeten your blood. These types of hyper-glycemic carbs send insulin soaring into the stratosphere, initiating an unstoppable anabolic force within your body that will store calories at an overwhelming rate, leading to excessive energy availability. And unless you're actively pounding out reps on a bench press, climbing a mountain, or running, the overabundance of energy will go straight to your ass. Literally.

The second step is to replace high-glycemic carbs with low-glycemic carbs. Low-glycemic carbohydrates will deliver the necessary energy for work, but with the minimalist side effects of insulin delivery. Because low-glycemic carbs are slow carbs, they minimally raise blood sugar, thus preventing sweet blood. Consequently, they trigger a minimal insulin response and thus take longer to deliver energy. Call it a trickle delivery energy system. Stable blood sugar and stable insulin equal manageable energy assimilation and use, therefore preventing overabundant energy that will more likely be used for work than stored as body fat.

Low-glycemic carbs are foods like beans, oats, brown rice, yams, couscous, and fibrous vegetables. These foods have a molecular makeup that takes longer for your digestive system to break down and assimilate. Fast carbs may take thirty minutes to two hours to go through your system, whereas slow carbs (low-glycemic carbs) take much longer, usually four to six hours, for your body to break down, assimilate, and use. Low-glycemic carbs may not have the overwhelmingly blissful tastes of high-glycemic carbs, they but will prevent energy crashes by providing sustained energy for work, play, sex, recreation, and more.

The Glycemic Index

How can you determine if a carbohydrate is high, low, or moderate glycemic? This is defined by a tool called the glycemic index. The glycemic index (GI) rates each carbohydrate on a scale from 0 to 100. Pure glucose is 100, and a baked potato has a GI of 85. Peanuts have a low rating of 14; bean sprouts and grapefruit have a GI of 25. The number or glycemic rating represents the blood sugar and subsequent insulin responses after consuming carbohydrates. The higher the number, the higher the blood sugar and insulin response. So, preventing sweet blood and insulin is simple: eat only low-glycemic carbohydrates or no carbs at all.

What do I mean by "no carbs at all"? Is this even possible?

Absolutely. In fact, this is something that lean, athletic, and health-conscious people do often. It's called carbohydrate fasting. Short-term fasting of all foods in general, called total fasting, has many health benefits, including improving blood sugar control, lowering blood insulin, reducing insulin resistance, lowering tissue inflammation, lowering your cholesterol, improving heart health, improving cognitive functioning, lowering the threshold for neurodegenerative disorders, promoting weight loss, boosting your metabolism, increasing growth hormone (which improves strength and thus performance), maximizing overall longevity, and preventing cancer. Bodybuilders and most athletes need their calories to maintain athletic performance, strength, and muscle mass. Therefore, they use carbohydrate fasting, otherwise referred to as carb depletion, to experience all the benefits of total fasting yet maintain the benefits of protein consumption.

What do you eat, then, if you eat no carbs at all?

To deplete carbs, you consume only meats (all types), fish, eggs, tofu, protein shakes, and other protein supplements (like Protein Puffs by Twin Peaks Ingredients). You can also modify carb fasting to your liking. During their EXERLEAN transformations, my clients use carb depletion to reach a state of glycogen depletion. This is referred to as *the State*. The State is when your body depletes glycogen and enters total body fat incineration. Glycogen is glucose stored in muscles to be used for work when needed. To completely abstain from sweet blood, you must first carb deplete, then carb deplete until muscle glycogen is depleted as well. This is when you enter ketosis: when the body has no energy from carbohydrates and muscle glycogen is depleted, it will start devouring its body fat stores to use for energy. People who follow a ketogenic diet maintain this state of ketosis and devour body fat by eating a high-protein and mild-to-moderate-fat diet, all while abstaining from any carbohydrates.

The EXERLEAN protocol for total body fat incineration does not fully deplete carbs and does not advocate a high-fat diet but rather a low-fat diet. The total body fat incinerator is a diet of high protein, moderate fibrous low-GI carbs, and low fat. Yet to reach the State of total body fat incineration, you must first carb deplete until all muscle glycogen is depleted and ketosis is reached, then you must start consuming a diet that's high protein, moderate low-calorie, fibrous low-GI carb, and low fat. Meat and veggies only; no bread, no pasta, no desserts, no sugar. By consuming low-GI "fibrous" carbs, you can stay just out of ketosis, which prevents muscle wasting and maintains the flame that metabolizes body fat like a Hoover vacuum at a confetti party.

The State: the fat-burning zone

The first step in the total body fat incinerator is to reach the State. This takes two to three days of strict carb depletion, usually with exercise, to fully eliminate muscle glycogen. Next, you add in daily low-GI and low-calorie fibrous carbs to bounce out of yet hover near ketosis. Hovering just out of ketosis, maintaining muscle glycogen depletion, and sustaining low blood sugar is the zone of maximal fat-burning potential. This is being in the State.

The total body fat incinerator: the fat-burning cycle

The second step in the total body fat incinerator is to maintain the State of maximal fat burning for four to nine days, depending on whether you are doing one- or two-week cycles of the total body fat incinerator algorithm. The third step is to prevent accommodation and confuse the body to keep your metabolism jacked. You do this by consuming a high-carbohydrate diet for one or two days. This is referred to as carbohydrate loading. In this day or two of carb loading, you eat carbs that are moderate GI and higher calorie, like beans, rice, pasta, fruit, and oats. This takes advantage of the anabolic burst cycle theory: if you fast and then gorge, your body cannot become habituated to a certain diet, thus keeping your metabolism and anabolism high, which preserves lean body mass and incinerates body fat. After one to two days of carb loading, it's back to square one: carb depletion to reach the State, a few days in the total body fat incinerator, then a short burst of carb loading, then repeat. This is the total body fat incinerator, the EXERLEAN diet algorithm created by me. Prepare to melt body fat off your carcass like never before and never again.

Obliterate body fat.

Obliterate sweet blood.

Two books can help you fully understand and achieve these objectives: *EXERLEAN* and The Total Body Fat Incinerator, both written by me. Get these books on Amazon, at Barnes & Noble, or from other bookstores and retailers.

Obliterate Sludge Blood

Sludge blood is fat- and cholesterol-saturated blood that results from routinely eating fatty foods, like french fries, pizza, churros, cheeseburgers, fatty meats, donuts, cookies, and any deep-fried foods. Cholesterol and fats you eat are converted to lipoproteins and triglycerides. Lipoproteins are spherical proteins otherwise known as high-density lipoproteins (HDL) or low-density lipoproteins (LDL). Triglycerides are made from glycerol and three fatty acids and are the main component of body fat.

Fat in the bloodstream is a good source of energy for work, but if you're sedentary, energy is not needed and will only increase the conversion of excess energy into additional body fat, or in the case of fat in the bloodstream, fat goes straight to fat. Having fat in your blood is a streamlined road to getting fatter without much work at all. Aside from the increased potential to store more body fat by consuming a high-fat diet, there are other consequences of having fat flowing through your veins and arteries. Elevated fat in your bloodstream puts you at high risk of developing atherosclerosis, or plaque accumulation on your artery walls. This plaque gets thicker and thicker over time and increases your risk of heart attacks, strokes, and cognitive decline.

Eating a diet high in saturated fats and trans fats leads to blood with high cholesterol. Cholesterol is a waxy substance that your body needs for cellular repair and growth. Cholesterol is carried through the bloodstream by attaching to proteins. The combination of cholesterol and proteins is called lipoproteins. Low-density lipoproteins (LDL) are considered the bad cholesterol, and high-density lipoproteins (HDL) are considered the good cholesterol. When LDL builds up on the arterial walls, it leads to hardened and narrow arteries. HDL helps collect excess cholesterol in the bloodstream and return it to the liver. Too much cholesterol puts you at risk of heart disease. High cholesterol leads to fatty deposits on blood vessel walls. These fatty deposits (plaques) continue to collect until they grow so large that they impair blood flow (atherosclerosis) and, in some cases, eventually close off circulation completely.

When I was in OT school, we had had a cadaver anatomy class in which three or four students completely dissected a human cadaver over the school year. When dissecting the cadaver's carotid arteries, I vividly remember seeing thick, hard inner linings of the carotids, the major blood vessels of the neck. This hard lining was whitish and felt like glass. I was able to snap a section like a long, thin piece of porcelain. It was a real face slapper to see and feel hardened arteries, with the hardness of glass yet the brittleness of porcelain, and a contrasting color from arterial tissue. This put the whole idea into perspective, that a piece of these can break off and go straight to the brain and cause a stroke. All from the buildup of unused fat in the blood.

Sludge blood puts you at high risk of obesity, kidney disease, high blood pressure, chest pain, heart attacks, and strokes. Your risk factors of experiencing these negative effects are higher if you are older, are overweight or obese, drink excessive alcohol, smoke cigarettes, eat an unhealthy diet, and don't exercise daily.

To obliterate sludge blood, you need to eat low-fat foods, stop smoking, minimize alcohol or abstain from it completely, start exercising daily, and prevent body fat accumulation for the rest of your life.

Obliterate Sedentary Behavior

"Oh, what a buzzkill," most fat and out-of-shape people would say at the mere thought of getting off their butts. Living in accordance with this attitude makes life grand and enjoyable, but it comes with long-term negative consequences. Sedentary behavior makes it too easy to succumb to pastimes—time spent in a suspended state of animation. Inanimate time spenders such as binge-watching TV, lounging around drinking beers, socializing at the club, playing bingo or cards, and going for a long drive. All these activities provide visual, auditory, olfactory, and emotional stimuli along the same lines as mood- and cognitive-enhancing drugs, but with less intensity. These activities are spent in sedentary time.

As you know by now, sedentary behavior is our tendency to avoid physical activity and remain in a state of sedentary time. Physical activity can cause pain, discomfort, pleasure, production of mood-enhancing endorphins, and physiological exhaustion. Sedentary time prevents all possibility of discomfort or pain from physical exertion. It is easy to develop a tendency to avoid the least amount of discomfort possible in exchange for maximal comfort. Remember, human instinct is to take the path of least resistance, and this path leads to negative physical and mental health consequences. The human body and mind need a challenge, need to experience some degree of pain and discomfort to gain and maintain physical strength and mental willpower. To develop pandemic armor and then keep it, you need to obliterate sedentary behavior and manage sedentary time strictly for rest and recovery from work.

Obliterate Negative Thoughts

Did you know that you can think yourself into sickness? You can crash your health and immunity if your mind is not fully engaged in a positive pathway. Your body is directly connected to your mind. Your thoughts influence your immunity. So, you can literally think yourself into susceptibility to illness and disease, even disability. Your thoughts can also promote improved health and wellness, enhancing your immunity. Positive thinking, confidence, and focus are the ingredients for a successful rocket launch and landing. Ever heard of the quote from success coach Brian Tracy, "You become what you think about most of the time"? Or the quote from author John Assaraf, "You attract what you think about most"? Or from radio speaker Earl Nightingale, "We become what we think about most of the time, and that's the strangest secret"? The idea is that in your life, you become and attract from the universe what you think about most of the time . . . and that's the strangest secret.

Here are some examples of some of the worst negative thought processes that will eat away at your soul and cool any possible positive and enlightening thoughts and feelings:

1. It doesn't matter.
2. Who cares?
3. It's just how it is.
4. If it wasn't for her . . .

5. It's not my fault.
6. I can't do it.
7. It's too late for me.
8. I'm not good enough.
9. That asshole.
10. Fyck him.
11. It's his fault.
12. It will never work.
13. I am this way because of . . .
14. I am a failure.
15. I am weak.

And on and on . . . you get the point. Just writing these negative thoughts down brings negative feelings, let alone conjuring them from within, actively thinking them, and then likely executing behaviors and actions from them throughout the day. A mindset focused on negativity conjures negative outcomes. The negative verbalizations listed here and similar thoughts go past the moment of creation. They pass through to your psyche, your soul, your emotions, finally resulting in your body experiencing the negative watershed effects of unhealthy catabolic and other depressing stress hormones caused by those negative thoughts. A negative thought process sends you down a negative path for the remainder of the day. That is not a day to look forward to, and lord have mercy on the people around you who will also be affected negatively by your radiating negativity. Negativity is contagious like a disease. It is a good thing, then, that positivity is also contagious, even counteracting negative energy. Smile. It delivers mind-blowing positive power. Motivational speaker Jim Rohn states that "we are the average of the five people we spend the most time with." Since this is so, surround yourself with positive, successful, and encouraging people, and your life will be so much better. So must you expel negative people—soul suckers—from your circle of five. You must obliterate all Karens, negative Nancys, and dickhead naysayers from your environment, or their repelling demeanors will rub off on you. You'll end up smelling like shit if you hang around it too long. And the shit will linger with you the rest of the day.

Positive thinking and focus bring self-control, happiness, and success. Surround yourself with similar-minded people, and you'll be so much better prepared for success.

Here are some examples of positive thinking that will put your mind, body, and soul in the realm of positivity and hope:

1. It matters to me.
2. I am surrounded by good people.
3. I am in control of my fate.
4. I take full responsibility for my present situation and the future.
5. I can do anything I put my mind to and pursue.
6. It's never too late so long as I am breathing.
7. I am successful.
8. She must be having a bad day; I wonder how I can help her?
9. God bless him with good fortune.
10. I am this way because of past actions, behaviors, thoughts, and the work I've accomplished.
11. I have a millionaire mind.
12. I am strong.
13. I am in control.
14. My thoughts, behavior, and actions are mine and mine alone, and therefore I accept full responsibility for everything that is my life.

15. Today I will turn that frown upside down; hug, care, give, be compassionate and show and feel gratitude.

These thoughts point you in the direction of positive movement. Negative thoughts do the opposite.

Take the story of a famous magazine entrepreneur who was in his younger years destined to be a failure. On the day the high school SAT scores were handed out, the teachers were stunned that he had a score of 1480 out of 1600. An SAT score represents a person's intelligence. People with high SAT scores live in the realms of Bill Gates, who scored 1590, Paul Allen (1600), and Rush Limbaugh (1530). According to the 2020 College Review Board annual report, the average SAT score is 1051. "Not possible," everyone was saying, including the boy's parents. "There is no way he can be that smart." But the boy swore up and down that he did not cheat.

Once the young man realized that he was smart, he decided to take more advanced classes and changed the crowd of kids he spent time with. People started to treat him like he was the smart person his score determined he was. He believed he was uber-smart and was behaving like it. After high school, he went on to an Ivy League college and ultimately became successful in the magazine business.

This story makes sense, right? A highly intellectual person is destined to become great. Well, this story has a twist. Twelve years after receiving his SAT score, the successful magazine entrepreneur received a letter from the Princeton University SAT review board explaining that thirteen students, including him, were accidentally sent the wrong SAT scores, and that his score was actually 740. That put his score in the bottom third percentile in the nation. Had he not been given the wrong SAT score in high school, though, he would not have believed he was ultra-smart, and his life may have gone in a different direction. His life changed the moment he believed he was smart and started acting like a smart person. His SAT score didn't determine whether he would be successful. Success is the result of optimism, perseverance, discipline, and work.

A negative past does not have to dictate your present behavior, actions, and goals. You control your thoughts, your behavior, your actions, and your verbalizations. "Think before you speak" is a well-known phrase because it is vital to verbalize what is necessary for communicating, uplifting yourself, and empowering others. When you get the urge to spit out some words, pause and take a second to decipher the words for meaning and content. Can the words be taken out of context? Can your tone or body language make someone want to repel away from you? Determine these things to deliver your message successfully and leverage the receiver's response to your desire.

Negative verbalizations are an extension of negative thoughts. You and you alone experience the negativity of your thoughts, but when you turn those thoughts into negative noise, you deal out your negative energy to everyone who can hear. Then they feel negativity. Obliterate negative verbal vomit. Nobody wants it, and ultimately negative thinking leads to lessened immunity.

Obliterate Complaining, Blaming, and Justification

There is no positive benefit to complaining. The goal of complaining is sympathy. Sympathy is a limited resource, and if you exhaust it from everyone around you, the well will run dry, and someday you'll find your complaining ass alone and avoided. Complaining might at first get you a dose of sympathy, but only once, maybe twice at the most.

Complaining mostly just pisses everyone off who has to endure it. This is not because people are mean or lack empathy; it is because we all have our problems, things we are worried about, and we just don't have much reserve capacity to endure someone else's problems. Complaining is something that a child does, often by whining and stomping their feet. Adults continue this childlike conduct with complaining, blaming, and justifying, which are advanced forms of immaturity, sciolism, and uncouthness. The next time you have to endure an adult complaining, take a mental step back and focus on what they are doing and how it is making you feel. Is it attractive? Does their complaining draw positive energy from you to share? It does not matter if there is any merit to the complaining; it never sounds or feels good coming out of an adult's mouth. At times, it may behoove you to give a dose of passive sympathy to a complainer so you can get away from this soul sucker.

Complaining is exercising your unhappiness or dissatisfaction about anything. Unconsciously, you think that doing so will help you feel better. But complaining does *not* help you feel better. How you respond to any predicament in life is 100 percent up to you, and complaining about it just pounds that seed of shit deeper into the earth, giving it a better chance at survival and spreading its roots out only to continue building the foundation of negativity that envelopes you and your experience of life.

Instead of complaining about something you are dissatisfied about, stop and breathe. Realize that what happened is already in the past and cannot be taken back. It cannot be changed. Whenever what was said or done that you are chapped about begins the inner churning of negative thoughts that you want to verbalize, do *not* share them. Remain in control of yourself. Can you think of a positive way to look at it? How can you learn from this? What can you do to make things better, because complaining won't accomplish anything positive? Smile. Say something positive. Take a positive step forward. Focus on your goals, and keep moving toward them.

The blame game, another immature tactic, attempts to repel a connection to something undesirable, like a failure or mistake, away from yourself. Know that so long as you breathe, you have control of how you experience your life and the shit, bad or great, that affects you. Instead of pointing the finger at something or someone else, turn the end of your pointer finger around toward your face. Whether it is on you or not, how you choose to think about it, feel about it, and react to it is 100 percent on you. Again, keep the power of control in your arsenal, because blaming gives your power of self-control to the external. Do you want to be controlled by others or have self-control?

Instead of blaming, take a moment to think about it. How can you turn this around in a positive and productive way? How can you choose to feel good rather than bad? Respond by harnessing the power of self-control, personal responsibility, and positive movement toward your goals. Your positive response will go noticed and will be felt by those around you, and magically the outcomes of your life will improve.

Obliterate Poor Self-Care

Remember that you must do a good job *caring* for yourself before you can tackle any higher-level skills in your life, like fighting off a dangerous predator or person, moving to safety, building shelter, hunting for food, caring for kids or elders, and contributing to the fabric of the community. If you're susceptible, weak, and unhealthy when a pandemic hits, you will not be able to do these things; you will be dependent on others. You must practice good self-care before even thinking of interviewing for a job. It is a given before you go out in public or get up close and personal with another person.

The outcomes and quality of your life stem from basic self-care, the quality and the level of how you perform basic human responsibilities. Your base human condition is a combination of how you care for your body, how well you control your thoughts and your emotions, and how well you do the work necessary for survival and living with purpose. When you have established a firm foundation in these basic life matters, you bolster your probability of success, and from this, you will garner maximum satisfaction with your life, learn and earn more, and ultimately maximize your immunity and pandemic armor.

Before we move on to the final letter in A.R.M.O.R., here are a few other things to obliterate that we've discussed before:

1. Smoking
2. Living in filth (your car, your house, and your work environment)
3. Excessive alcohol consumption (abstinence is the only guarantee in avoiding the negative effects of alcohol)
4. Nutritional deficiencies (take a multivitamin, eat colorful vegetables, and protein supplements)
5. Negative external influences (naysayers, pessimists, and complainers)
6. Eating directly before going to bed (practicing fasted sleep)
7. Bingeing TV, social media, and other addictions on the Internet of Things

"R"
RESOLUTION

*Always bear in mind that your own resolution to succeed is more
important than any other one thing. —Abraham Lincoln*

*No one's ever achieved financial fitness with a January
resolution that's abandoned by February. —Suze Orman*

Resolution is the final stage of developing your pandemic armor, the completion of your journey to harnessing the power of maximum immunity. There are many different definitions and ways to use the word *resolution*. We are focusing on two specific definitions. The first is the resolution to *resolve* an issue: to wrap up the journey of pandemic armor and achieve maximum immunity. The second deals with the most important element in your mission to develop pandemic armor: obliterating body fat. Just as a TV can change resolution or clarity so you can see the image better, weight loss and body fat incineration clear up the image of your body composition so you can see and feel what you're meant to look like. Body fat is blurring out the real image of you, and your primary mission in achieving your pandemic armor and maximum immunity is to get lean. Just like a New Year's resolution can resolve a problem over time, you can declare your new mission in life as a resolution to burn off all the body fat covering up your lean and muscular physique to maximize the resolution on the image of the physical you.

Starting right now, you must make a resolution to get lean, strong, and healthy. It is time to try new things. With new things comes new opportunity. Unless you are lean, strong, and immune, what you have been doing is not improving your health, so change is necessary—sometimes radical change, a full 180-degree switch-up, and an untraveled path to new beginnings.

As I've said before, to get lean, strong, and healthy, you must first *stop getting fatter*. Stop any further accumulation of body fat. This is easy to accomplish by making sure you are eating fewer calories than you burn off in a day.

Second, *build muscle*. Muscle mass or lean body mass is only a good thing. The leaner your body mass, the higher your metabolism, the stronger your immunity, and the more things you can physically conquer in life. This is easy to accomplish with a resistance training program, at home or at a gym. Lack of lean body mass leads to sarcopenia. Remember, sarcopenia is the result of protein starvation and muscle wasting as you age, leaving you gaunt, weak, frail, and immunocompromised. This is easy to prevent. Just make sure you are eating enough high-quality, high biological value protein every day.

Third, *stop smoking*. Smoking leads to susceptibility, poor health, low quality of life, and early death. There is nothing fundamentally easier to do than just stopping. Go cold turkey.

Fourth, *stop alcoholism*. Excess alcohol consumption leads to addiction, organ disease, cognitive impairment, poor quality of life, and early death. This again is easy to do by just abstaining!

Finally, *stop taking drugs*. Stop abusing any prescription drugs and using illicit drugs to easily win better health.

These five main things are all preventable. In the mission to survive and live a high-quality life filled with health and wellness, you must maximize your immunity from sickness, disease, and disability. To start, you need to make your resolutions evident, obvious, and covenantal. Make a specific plan to obliterate these five preventable immunocompromisers, do the work, and never stop until you're free from all five. You must be resolute. You must get shit done. When you become body-fat-free, smoke-free, alcohol-free, drug-free, muscular, and strong, you are wearing pandemic armor.

A low-resolution body is smooth, rounded, and blurred, and the more body fat you have, the more blurred you become. A high-resolution body is so muscular and chiseled that you can tell where each muscle is, where the most superficial arteries are located, the separation between each body part, and striations when you flex a muscle. A low-resolution body has rounded cheeks, a double chin, fat rolls, and big ankles. You cannot see any arteries or veins on a low-resolution body. A high-resolution body has six-pack abs, chiseled facial features, apparent circulating healthy arteries and veins, muscular bellies, and bony prominences wrapped in thin skin.

In a year and a half now of working the COVID-19 frontlines, I have never seen a high-resolution person in the hospital. Not one. We only see low-resolution physiques in their deathbeds on the frontline. The rest of the hospital is also predominantly reserved for low-resolution people. Healthy, lean people do not need hospitals.

In this final stage of A.R.M.O.R., we are going to combine the two definitions of resolution to one simple definition of our goal. As we walk away from this book, we are going to become resolute in our mission to survive. To make the necessary resolutions in the game of life, which is leveraged toward survival of the fittest and living in a high-resolution body.

To win this game, we need to change our unhealthy habits, our body composition, and our mindsets. To eliminate the negative attributes that lead to poor health, disease, and disability. To do this, we start by making a resolution to achieve pandemic armor and maximum immunity. New Year's is the most common time to start on a mission to lose weight, stop smoking, abstain from alcohol, start working out, and live free from addiction. A resolution can start at any time, though. For the sake of you and everyone you care about, declare your resolution and start it now. There will never be a better time to get shit done. The past is dead, and the future depends on you. You make you the way you are and the way you will be.

Now, make your New Year's resolutions to get a high-resolution body. Envision the way a healthy person looks and feels . . . a high-resolution physique, muscles for work, managed energy, the ability to participate in recreation, seven hours of sleep, and seventeen hours of living a day. Resolve to become a healthy person with a beautiful, lean physique, endless energy, great sleep, and physical fitness. Write your resolutions down. Come up with a start date, then execute on schedule. Take notes or keep a journal along the way. Keep track of your weight, body part measurements, feelings, and failures. Seek expert counsel when needed. Hire a personal trainer to learn how to navigate and master exercising at a gym. Seek help from your primary care physician in your mission to lose weight, quit smoking, abstain from alcohol, limit prescription drugs, abstain from illicit drugs, and add lean body mass. Pick a diet plan to follow, and stick with it.

I recommend abstaining from television in your resolutions to change. As part of my evaluation when I first see a hospital patient, I ask, "What do you do in your spare time? What do you do for fun?" Nine out of ten times, the answer is "watch TV." Remember, we do not see healthy, lean people in the hospital, not for preventable admits. Healthy, lean people rarely go to a hospital, and it is usually by choice to get a joint replacement or other health-enhancing treatment or procedure. Unhealthy people are admitted to the hospital to prevent death from, for the most part, preventable predicaments. The frequent flyers to hospitals are overweight or obese, smokers or former smokers, drug abusers or former drug abusers, deconditioned and out of shape, noncompliant to medical advice, and not exercising frequently, if ever. Their lives are the results of years and years of continued unhealthy choices and indolent behavior. Their bodies are so out of shape that they are uncomfortable doing physical activity or recreation, so they end up watching television as the only means of entertainment and leisure. If you stop watching TV, your chances of finding something physically healthy to do increase.

CONCLUSION

You now have the necessary ingredients for maximizing your immunity and wearing pandemic armor. The C.A.R.E. and A.R.M.O.R. algorithms will lead you on the fastest path from susceptibility to pandemic armor and maximum immunity. Pandemic armor is a program in action, execution, and perseverance. The simple action steps you can initiate right now are:

1. **Stop adding body fat.** Decrease your daily food intake. Don't worry about what kind of diet you are going to go on right now. Just eat less. Simple things you can do to lower your calorie intake are to eliminate calorie-dense hyperpalatable foods. Stop eating all sweets, including chocolate. Switch from any coffee shop drink to coffee, espresso, or tea with no milk, creamers, or sweeteners. Simply eliminating these things will start you on the road to weight maintenance and, when you are ready to start a weight loss program, the road to fasting and total body fat incineration.

2. **Stop smoking.** Go cold turkey. Smoking is not like food. You cannot wean yourself from smoking and be healthy. Even one cigarette is damaging your lungs. Just quit. Don't smoke anything!

3. **Eat more protein.** This is the simple answer to preventing and treating sarcopenia. Replace fats and carbs with high biological value protein sources like lean beef, fish, chicken, turkey, eggs, calcium caseinate, soy protein isolate, and whey. Humans need protein to build new cells, build muscle, feed the body, and foster maximum immunity.

4. **Stop consuming alcohol.** Alcoholism is preventable and treatable. Excessive alcohol leads to obesity, diabetes, kidney and liver disease, and a decline in brain function. There is no nutritional benefit to alcohol. Most alcoholic beverages are high glycemic, are high in empty calories, promote sweet blood, and can lead to addiction. I bet you that most people would admit that the situations they regret most in life and wish to undue involved alcohol. Alcohol gives you a firsthand introduction to shit you will regret for the rest of your life. In your journey to maximize your immunity and survive a pandemic, abstaining from or at least minimizing your alcohol intake is the best choice.

5. **Say no to drugs.** Overconsumption and addiction to painkillers are some of the top preventable causes of death in adults around the world. There is no benefit to taking drugs to numb awareness of feelings and sensations. This is the road to addiction and early death.

Who succeeds in life is based on one simple thing: obliterating the top five susceptibilities. The most immune and successful people in life do not even contemplate activities or thoughts that will possibly hinder their goals of health, wellness, and wealth. Being fat, smoking, and doing drugs are not options. You can drastically leverage your chances of accomplishing anything you want purely by abstaining from bad shit. Want to up the ante? Do the shit people are too lazy, fearful, or otherwise hesitant to do, and do it with extreme passion, then finish strong. Spend more time doing things that matter, and make gains toward your goals step-by-step, replacing things that don't matter. Spend your time doing what will inevitably make a positive difference in your life. By preventing the bad in life, you can leverage your chances of happiness, health, and wealth. This is a simple fact of life. Because when you eliminate all the bad, only good remains.

AFTERWORD

People, I love you. I want the best this world and your body have to offer you. I have felt over and over the true awesomeness of walking around in a super-lean and muscular physique, all the while having real belief in self. When you are lean, light, and strong, eat lean, and focus on positivity, life is so good. It is real and achievable to every living human being, on every continent, at any age. Living with pandemic armor and maximum immunity is the dream. With pandemic armor, you will survive when shit hits the fan.

I rarely get sick, and when I do get sick, it is because I am putting myself on the frontline and exposing myself to sick people. You deserve maximum immunity. You deserve to survive. You can eliminate the negative and adopt the positive. You control you. You can lose *all* the body fat and be super lean, entering the 1 percent of super-awesome human existence. When you feel it and walk around in it, you will know this is the magic. This is what a human is meant to feel. This is how a human is supposed to live. There are no self-induced restrictions that are the "benefits" of obesity, poor self-care, addiction, and indolent behavior. Only the benefits of work, of physical strength, of following your passion, of walking around in a lean body, of living with pandemic armor, and of having the personal security of maximum immunity. You can achieve anything you set your mind to if you follow your path and show up every day to the fight for personal achievement. Never give up on the pursuit of maximal health, wellness, and survivability.

BONUS MATERIAL

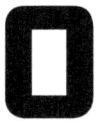

One chapter from each book of the EXERLEAN Transformation Trilogy, a series designed to help you get in the best shape of your life and achieve maximum immunity

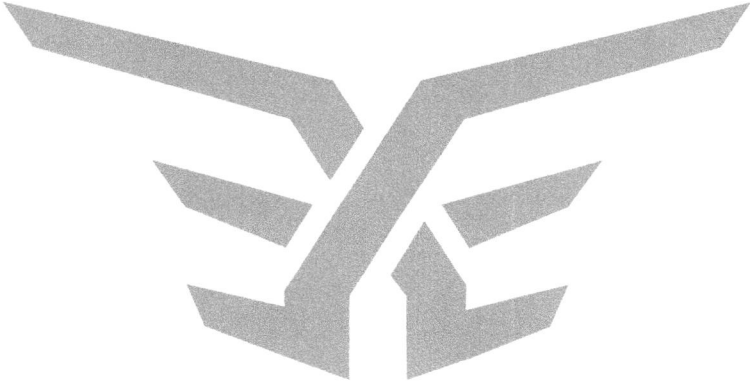

EXERLEAN

TEASER 1
EXERLEAN

CONTENTS

CHAPTER 1
THE FACE SLAP

Are you sick and tired of living unhealthy, feeling like a low-energy pile of crap, and never being able to see beyond the fat on your body every time you look in the mirror? Well, look no further because this book, right here in your hands, has everything necessary to help you put an end to excess body fat and the negative consequences that come with it.

Before you read any further, I want to warn you that this book is a slap-in-the-face, no-holds-barred, possibly-some-bad-words *awakening*.

An awakening to the reality of the world around you and why the majority of people are overweight, sedentary, and in some cases, dying earlier than they should. You may be one of them!

Okay, now . . . if you're complaining, then pull up your big-boy or big-girl pants and accept that you may be part of the worldwide obesity epidemic.

Hold on to your saddlebags! We are about to take a ride down reality lane.

"Let's Do This!"

Two out of three adult human beings are considered overweight, obese, or morbidly obese as of 2018 per the National Institutes of Health (NIH). Per 2013–2014 NHANES (National Health and Nutrition Examination Survey) data, **70.2 percent of adults are overweight or obese, 32.5 percent are overweight, and 37.7 percent are obese, of which 7.7 percent includes extreme obesity**. Additionally, **three out of four men** (73.7 percent) and **two out of three women** (66.9 percent) **are considered overweight, obese, or morbidly obese**. Sadly, **one in six youth** ages two to nineteen (17.2 percent) were considered to be obese (NHANES Data, NIH).

Now I'm not saying you're overweight, but your chances of being overweight or obese are overwhelming. Most of us are overweight at the minimum. In fact, unless you have been on and are currently undergoing some sort of exercise routine and have been eating lean, then you are at a minimum overweight and possibly obese.

So, from here forward knowing that over 70 percent of us are overweight, obese, or morbidly obese, we have a literally big problem on our hands. Unless you're in the less than 30 percent of people maintaining a healthy weight, then you desperately need to take everything this book has to offer, cram it down your throat, and live it out.

Let the awareness of the obesity epidemic move you toward a positive change. To help you on your journey to lose weight, get strong, and learn and adopt healthy, lean living habits.

I call this a transformation of a person's *healthstyle*. Lifestyle includes everything about you and how you're living—your car, job, hobbies, religion, beliefs, morals, activities, routines, schedules, health, exercise, etc. Your healthstyle includes everything you engage in mentally, physically, leisurely, and workwise that actually and factually dictates your current state of body composition, health, and wellness.

Moving forward, we are going to talk about some possibly shocking, personal, and revealing details about humanity that may initially offend you, maybe humiliate you, possibly upset you. But fear not—there is a greater mission than that at hand.

After assimilating the knowledge, statistics, and resources this book offers, the goal is that you will become externally influenced and internally motivated for positive change. To change your ways, to stake your claim on this earth and make your life the best it can be.

**"Anything can happen if you make a move.
Nothing different will if you don't." —Me**

In 2004, while in the school of occupational therapy (OT) at Eastern Washington University (EWU), I wrote a research paper and grant application to the National Institutes of Health titled, "Does Obesity Affect a Person's Occupational Performance in Community Mobility?" The results of my study were staggering. One of the first things I became aware of from my research was the exponential rising prevalence of obesity in America, especially in children. As to my research title's question, the overwhelming statistics and data reveal the answer is a huge yes. Sadly, obesity does negatively affect a person's ability to mobilize within their community and the quality of their mobilization. For example, these problems could include requirements to pay for two airplane seats due to buttocks width, use of power scooters for shopping, inaccessibility through standard-width doorways, higher-priced furniture and medical equipment to handle the excess weight, and difficulty getting on and maneuvering public buses or subway systems. The list goes on and on and on.

Sadly, since I did that research at OT school in 2004, the obesity epidemic is only growing exponentially out of control. Straight to who knows where. At the rate that body fat is increasing in the United States, we are headed toward a 100 percent overweight and obese population.

Why the trend?

What's the reason for the epidemic of overweight people?

CHAPTER 2
THE OBESIBOOMERS

What we are seeing and dealing with all started with the silent generation of the early 1900s, specifically 1925 to 1942 during the ramping up of automotive technology and air travel. This is when the flash flood of market-to-consumer products began. High-tech luxuries to make our lives easier. Cars, motorcycles, airplanes, and public transportation systems. No more horses, walking, or riding bikes as a necessity.

The baby boomers' post–World War II generation from about 1940 to 1964 on to Generation X of 1960 to 1981 to the millennial generation and now Generation Z have all reaped the exponentially accumulating benefits of scientific and industrial breakthroughs. We are now living in the splendor and bliss of the technological age. The environment around us makes this undeniable! We are living in the easiest, least physically demanding, most plentiful, and most accessible time in human history.

Easy access to foods, drinks, transportation, and sedentary work environments are at an all-time high and rising with the continual advances in science and technology. And with it, we as a human race have become overweight, obese, and sedentary. Welcome to the dawn of the Obesiboomers!

It's undeniable that we as humans are in a booming phase in the evolution of our species, similar to the massive spike in baby births mid-twentieth century that gave rise to the term *baby boomers*. Well, our species is undergoing a massive transformation into the nether realm of obesity, obesity-related diseases, and obesity-related disabilities. The Obesiboomer epidemic is not specific to one generation, race, or county. Obesity does not discriminate. It is a trend involving the majority of the world. With rates of three out of four U.S. adults being either overweight or obese, the odds are in favor of 70 percent of all people around you being overweight or obese, including yourself. As I said earlier, one in six children are obese, a trend that is only rising and showing no signs of a downtrend or stabilization. This leads in only one direction as we head into the future. A surge in the Obesiboomer epidemic.

The Walt Disney movie *WALL·E* paints a great vision into the future of mankind and how technology may become so advanced that machines will do everything for us. If you haven't seen the movie, I highly recommend watching it as soon as you can. It is a rewarding film for all ages. To sum up the part I am referring to, basically humans live in an automated community on the massive spaceship the *Axiom*. The *Axiom* is so automated that the residents don't even have to walk. They float everywhere they need to go in little hover chairs, enjoying food in overabundance and entertainment galore. They are extremely sedentary, and consequently, everybody is morbidly obese.

This could be the future of the human race if sedentary human behavior becomes the norm and technological advancements keep simplifying our ability to work or not work.

The Obesiboomer millennia is birthed from an environment of less and less physical work. We as a human race are engaging in less and less physically exerting activity as technology makes our lives easier. To fix this dilemma, we need to add in physical work or exercise to compensate for the lack of exertion taking place. The human body needs physical work, exertion, and weight-bearing activity every day to maintain skeletal integrity, muscle functions, and body composition.

Bones need bone-on-bone pressure and weight-bearing activity to stay strong, otherwise sedentary behavior and lack of that pressure will lead to bone demineralization, decreased bone density, mechanical destabilization, and possible structural deformity over time.

Muscles need work and force to maintain mass and strength. Lack of necessary workload on muscles leads to the pruning of muscle tissue and muscle atrophy. This muscle wasting in turn leads to weaker muscle functions, low energy, and lower metabolism.

Without daily workload, our body composition (the balance or ratio between muscles, body fat/adipose tissue, and bone) is distorted away from our natural healthy state of being. Body fat increases, lean body tissue or muscle decreases, and bones become smaller and frail. Add to that, if we are not physically active doing something, then we must consequently be doing nothing—likely sitting in a chair, reading this book, or watching television. Then, human behavior, boredom, and bad habits take over; we grab a snack and start eating garbage at the same time we're being sedentary. This leads to even more body fat storage.

You know the story.

Obesity is preventable and treatable. The chapters to come will provide you with all the right information you need to take control of yourself and your actions.

To take a stand against sedentary behavior and the overstuffing of our faces. To get out of the fat race.

CHAPTER 3
WHY CHANGE?

Before we get into the secrets on how to change your ways, your health, and your body composition, we first need to fully understand the why.

Why change?

I mean, what's so bad about being overweight or obese? It's the new norm, it's accepted, and as time goes by, it's universally rationalized or even normalized as beautiful and healthy. Nobody really cares if you're overweight or obese.

What does it matter?

Is media and societal-driven propaganda coaxing or forcing us to accept being overweight or obese as normal, beautiful, or good?

I've never heard someone say that "her folds of fat and cratered cellulite legs are really flattering." or "Oh, boy, he's got an attractive, bulbous potbelly."

I mean, come on, let's stick to reality here. You'd be living a lie if you said or tried to convince yourself that folds of fat, dimply legs, or protruding potbellies were attractive, preferred, or normal compared to a slender, muscular, or lean physique.

"Come on, everyone's doing it."

Does a societal norm make something a good thing just because the majority are experiencing it, like obesity?

Yeah, let's all jump off the cliff.

If it's not good, then it must be bad, and if it's bad . . . how bad? How bad is being overweight, obese, or morbidly obese . . . really?

Okay, well, where do we start? Let's start with this: the most up-to-date information from the NIH and the Centers for Disease Control and Prevention (CDC). Obesity and obesity-related diseases lead to early death.

Death!

Yes, dead before your time. In other words, people who are not overweight or obese stand a much greater chance at longevity than fat people. Add to this, the last decade or two of life is of much lower quality for obese or morbidly obese persons. This is due to their poor health status, poor ability to self-care, joint destruction, poor mobility, and onset of and living with obesity-related diseases and disabilities.

I have worked as an occupational therapist (OT) since 2004 in the acute care hospital setting with direct patient care. I'm the guy who comes into a patient's room and helps them get out of bed, mobilize, and engage in self-care. OTs focus on helping people rehabilitate from surgery, illness, disease, or disability. We do this by facilitating their engagement in self-care and mobility, as well as quality of life. We initiate exercises or therapeutic activities to get people up and moving so they can take care of themselves and return to their home.

I've helped thousands of patients rehabilitate and continue to do so full time. As an OT in an acute care hospital setting, I see everything. I work with people going through negative life events including intubation on a ventilator in the intensive care unit (ICU), strokes and heart attacks, pneumonia, falls with injury, trauma from motor vehicle accidents, and respiratory failure. I bounce all over the hospital, from the oncology unit to cardiac to the ER to the mental health ward and the surgical unit. My job is to teach people how to live after a neck, back, hip, knee, or any other surgery.

I've seen thousands of different diseases, disabilities, trauma situations, and other various physical or mental defects and intervene to help people deal with these problems so they can recover, take care of themselves, and move on in their lives. Much of the stuff people live with is truly unbelievable.

As Winston from the original *Ghostbusters* movie put it, "I've seen shit that will turn you white!"

Healthcare workers see firsthand how people deal with and recover from sickness, disease, or traumatic events. Ask any acute care therapist or nurse, and they will tell you that morbid obesity is one of the most disabling and unhealthy states of human existence. It affects absolutely everything in a negative way.

In order to develop the inner power necessary to make real physical, mental, and lifestyle changes, you need to know the *why*. The knowledge of why gives you the power to change. Then you can enter the battle against obesity. You need to have full knowledge of why you're in the fight against obesity, why body fat is your enemy, and why your life depends on winning the war.

The truth behind being overweight or obese is much more involved than just people being larger, having health problems, and likely dying earlier than expected. The obvious and well-publicized *negative effects* of obesity are prevalent.

Here is a summary of obesity-related data taken from the CDC website: "People who have obesity, compared to those with a normal or healthy weight, are at increased risk for many serious diseases and health conditions, including the following:"

Wait, let's stop there for a second. Before going into the details of these negative effects, I want to point out that government entities like the CDC, universities, and other research entities use very careful language and water down the verbiage to speak about the effects of obesity, choosing words like "are at increased risk," "associated with obesity," "may contribute." I will tell you straight up based on my years of clinical experience and treating people with obesity that obese people absolutely experience and endure more diseases, disabilities, and serious health conditions than lightweight lean people. Some deal with a few too many afflictions at the same time.

Based on clinical observations, the older an obese person gets, the more diseases, health problems, and disabilities just keep piling up like a stack of pancakes. The next thing they know, they are suffering from multiple major issues, which greatly decreases their quality of life. Unfortunately, most obese people choose to deal with these negative effects rather than do anything to combat them.

So let us keep the language real. The CDC's list of obesity-related health disparities include:

All causes of death (mortality). Yes, death means dead. Obesity leads to dead people, or being dead sooner than later.

High blood pressure. Hypertension can quietly destroy your body, leading to strokes, blood clots, dementia, heart attacks, heart and kidney disease, anxiety, poor quality of life, disability, and even fatality. There it is again, death!

High LDL cholesterol (the bad cholesterol), low HDL cholesterol (the good cholesterol), and high levels of triglycerides (bad). Too much bad cholesterol leads to strokes, heart disease, peripheral artery disease (PAD), and various other health ailments. Not enough of the good cholesterol leads to heart disease, digestion problems, and other health ailments.

Coronary heart disease. The heart is the core of all things blood. It is the only pump in the body. When the pumping stops . . . life stops. Heart disease is the most common cause of death for adults in the US. A diseased heart or circulatory system leads to heart failure, heart attack, stroke, pulmonary embolism, aneurysm, peripheral artery disease, heart arrythmias, angina, and lower quality of life.

Type 2 diabetes. Don't blow this one off, it's horrible! Type 2 diabetes increases a person's risk of leg, finger, or hand amputations and of developing low vision, peripheral neuropathy (brain and spinal cord nerve damage), and kidney failure. This can lead to dependency on dialysis machines to live.

Gallbladder disease. Gallbladder disease involves abdominal pain, nausea and vomiting, and infections that can lead to needing surgery to remove the gallbladder—a high-risk surgery.

Osteoarthritis. Osteoarthritis is the breakdown of cartilage and bone within a joint. When you're walking around in public, you'll observe many obese people whose knees are bent inward and are touching each other. Many overweight and obese people have deformed knees and hips because our joints are not designed to handle all that excess weight, and as a result, they will fall apart and disintegrate over time without exercise. This leads to needing joint replacement surgery or living in pain, thus eventually becoming immobile and dependent on power scooters and wheelchairs.

Sleep apnea and breathing problems (drowning in fat). Don't overlook this one! I see it every day in the hospital. Many obese and morbidly obese people have to wear a CPAP (continuous positive airway pressure) or BiPAP (bilevel positive airway pressure) breathing-assist device to keep their airways opened because they are blocked by fat tissues. These people cannot tolerate lying in a normal bed, so the head of the bed needs to be elevated or propped up so they won't suffocate or drown in their own body mass.

Some cancers. All cancer is bad, and you should make every effort to decrease your risk of getting it.

Dementia. Studies have shown that high levels of belly fat are linked to higher levels of brain atrophy (shrinking brains) and dementia. According to a 2008 Massachusetts General Hospital study, heavier people have smaller brains. Obese people were found to have 8 percent smaller-than-average brains and also looked sixteen years older. It also found that people with the most belly fat between the ages of forty and forty-five are three times more likely than normal-weight people to develop dementia in their later years.

Low quality of life (QOL). Of all the negative effects of obesity, except for maybe increased risk of death, this one cannot be understated.

As we live out our existence, it is in our nature to seek out our best quality of life. Obesity is a detrimental weapon working against you on this journey. Long-term obesity leads to poor quality of life. Based on my clinical observations and working firsthand to help people living with obesity, it is never a good thing. I have never witnessed a benefit of obesity in my practice.

People living with obesity get accustomed to it and lose track of the difference between living with a healthy body weight and being heavy. They forget about being able to walk for miles, sitting in one airplane seat, being able to walk down the aisle of a bus without their thighs bouncing off each seat they pass, or walking straight through a narrow doorway versus having to go through sideways. This list is never-ending. All aspects of human life are negatively affected by obesity.

Stroke. We all know strokes are bad and can be disabling. As an OT, I work with victims of strokes and help them return to independent self-care and functional mobility. I help people strengthen the weak body parts affected by the stroke, and I help them return to their best possible lives.

Trust me on this one—obese and morbidly obese people with strokes are usually much worse off than a lightweight stroke victim. Unless it's a minor stroke or a stoke that clears fast, obese people are screwed. Not only do they lose half their body function, but the remaining unaffected overweight side of the body has to carry around its weight and all the weight of the overweight paralyzed side. Add to that, most people with obesity live sedentary lives and are therefore deconditioned in the first place.

Nurses and therapists working with obese and morbidly obese people have their work cut out for them. They are at high risk of injury due to the excess burden of care an obese person requires. In many cases, nurses and therapists must use power cranes to move obese people in and out of bed to a commode or wheelchair. On the contrary, nonobese people are lighter and work less to self-care and mobilize, even with severe stroke deficits. Lightweight people have a much better chance of being able to get in and out of bed or transfer with caregiver assistance and without a crane.

Obese people in the hospital require heavy-duty specialty beds, wheelchairs, and bedside chairs to hold their weight. It's much more expensive, time consuming, and difficult to care for an obese or morbidly obese person compared to a healthy-weight person in the hospital setting. Many obese stroke sufferers end up in nursing homes for the rest of their lives. Healthy and lighter-weight people have much better odds of being able to return home or move to a lesser-care environment than a nursing home.

Family including spouses have a much better chance at being able to help you at home or take care of you if you are healthy and lightweight. Many patients and their families cannot afford the heavy-duty equipment necessary to care for obese and morbidly obese people. In many cases, they are forced to quit their jobs so they can be at home all the time to meet an obese person's higher-care needs. This is one of the reasons nursing homes have a high prevalence of obese residents. Most families cannot handle all that massive weight, give up their jobs, afford the heavy-duty furniture, or give up all their time to care for obese people with severe disability.

There is no going back. The ability to exercise is greatly diminished after a stroke with obesity, and therefore the ability to exercise and lose weight is more difficult. Restrictive dieting is basically the only option at this point, and I can tell you straight up that I've never seen a morbidly obese person with a disability change their behavior and diet to lose all that extra weight to make self-care and mobility easier, not one case in sixteen years. A lifetime of bad eating behavior is not easy to break, although it is absolutely possible. If you are obese, the time to take action is now, not later. Do it now before you stroke out!

Mental illness. Mental illness includes clinical depression, anxiety, and other mental disorders. If you had to live with half the stuff mentioned so far, how could you remain truly happy? We have the power to control how we feel, yes, but you must admit, these ailments would be very difficult to live with twenty-four hours a day and remain mentally unscathed, not to even mention the dissatisfaction with your appearance.

Body pain. What I predominantly see in my practice is that obese people have a much higher prevalence of spine, hip, knee, and ankle pain. Almost all obese people deal with cellulitis, a predicament when their skin gets infected and starts blowing up with puss-oozing fluids. Cellulitis is highly painful and hypersensitive. It usually requires antibiotics to treat. Not all, but most patients with fibromyalgia that I have come in contact with are overweight or obese. Fibromyalgia is another painful infliction.

Now here's where we are going to get down to the nitty-gritty, the behind-the-scenes situations that healthcare workers see firsthand:

How obesity affects personal care.

CHAPTER 4
WIPE YOUR OWN!

Let's cut to the chase and reveal the stuff people don't talk about when it comes to obesity. The most personal and intimate areas of our lives that are taboo to discuss. Personal to the core.

In addition to all the health problems we've mentioned, obesity and especially morbid obesity negatively affect personal self-care. Some obvious effects include difficulty getting in and out of bed, decreased walking distance, difficulty climbing up and down stairs, struggling to get in and out of a car, decreased productivity at work or inability to work, lower energy, and on and on. You can't push a marble through a pinhole.

We never openly discuss our personal abilities to self-care. Think about it. When is the last time you talked to someone about the quality of your ability to brush your teeth or cut your toenails? When's the last time you talked about the quality of your bathing and ability to reach every nook and cranny? "Hey, Bertha! Are you able to get your socks and shoes on these days?" Conversations like this just don't happen openly until self-care is an issue.

It's weird to think that people have difficulty with self-care. For the geriatric population, this is expected at some point as the body ages, becomes frail, and eventually closes in on the end of its days.

Self-care can also be challenging for those with disability from congenital or birth defects, traumatic disability, and injury from accident or other trauma. These issues are accidental and sometimes unpreventable. What we are talking about here is people who are afflicted with the preventable state of being overweight, obese, and morbidly obese.

As we discussed earlier, healthcare workers see thousands and thousands of people daily, many living with obesity and in desperate situations of self-care failure. Much of what they see in the hospital would turn you white, ghost white! They know firsthand the raw truth about how obesity affects people's ability to take care of themselves.

If you're not a nurse, therapist, doctor, or other medical team member, then you're likely just seeing obese people from their outside appearance, walking around, dressed, living life. You would never know or suspect what we are about to talk about based on outward appearances unless you are already living with these problems.

Let's start with a basic activity we do every day and sometimes multiple times a day: getting dressed.

Imagine not being able to dress yourself. We take this basic daily event for granted, and not a second thought goes to it. We just wake up and at some point put our clothes on. Well, for many obese people, it isn't that easy.

The ability to get dressed is all attributed to basic body mechanics. Arms and legs are only so long, and our bodies are designed to freely bend over, reach, and move. It's obvious that at some point, the sheer volume of body fat will decrease a person's range of motion and structurally block the hand from being able to reach the foot. The thick fat layers at the abdomen and thighs smashing up against each other leads to the inability to bend normally and with limited limb flexibility. Lower-body dressing is the first to go—socks, pants, shoes, and yes, even underwear.

"What?" you might be asking. "You mean people are walking around underwearless?" Yeah, man, it's quite common. Many are also sockless, with slip-on shoes, sandals, or slippers. Take a look next time you're out and about. Why are so many obese people wearing sandals, flip-flops, or slippers . . . in the frickin' winter? Because most are physically not able to put on socks and tie shoes anymore.

You say, "The obese and morbidly obese people I encounter in public are not able to get dressed?" Well, there is a workaround to this dressing dilemma. Adaptive equipment can increase a person's ability to reach their lower body. You know, those long-handled sticks with a trigger at one end and a claw at the other, usually referred to as a "reacher" or a "grabber." A person can use one of those or a dressing stick to claw the waistband of underwear and pants, then with the increased length or reach provided by the stick, thread the garments over the feet and pull them up to a point where the other hand can finally physically grasp the waistband (usually at knee level) and yank it the rest of the way up. Socks can be slipped on with a tool called a sock aid, a three-fingered foldable device on two long ropes that allows you to stuff a sock on to it, flip it down to your feet, and with the two ropes yank the sock on over your foot. What about shoes? Well, laces are difficult to tie with a stick. You can add elastic laces and pretie them, but this is time consuming, so most obese people just wear slip-on shoes, flip-flops, or sandals.

This sounds like a lot of work, huh? Most obese patients I work with wear slip-on shoes and loose, baggy clothing. So loose they can whip the waistband down and thread it over their feet. Many just wear a single-piece nightgown or muumuu—and not because it's the new cool style! This dressing style is out of necessity. All that extra mass is a structural blockade between the upper body and the lower body. When it comes down to it, many obese people get their spouses, significant others, or kids to help them get dressed and avoid using adaptive equipment altogether because it's easier just to let someone else do it.

This mind-blowing knowledge must be enough to thrust your motivation train into high gear. I bet you're standing up, doing jumping jacks, or performing some other exercise right now. Right? No. Not yet. You're not feeling it. You don't care that much about getting yourself dressed or what clothing you wear. But maybe you're a bit provoked or intrigued? Okay, well, let's keep the momentum going. Let's keep that motivation train running and add fuel to the fire. We haven't even gotten into bathing yet!

"Oh, no! Not bathing. Please tell me differently," you're saying to yourself. Well, sorry—there is a reason BO (body odor) is common among people with a lot of extra body fat. For one, there is much more square footage of excretion tissue (how the skin releases oils, sweat, and toxins), and if the skin is rolling or folding up on itself, then things in the darkness cannot breathe. This sounds like a line in a horror movie. Well, take a sniff of fresh BO, and you'll feel like you're the superstar smack dab in the middle of a horror movie yourself.

It is difficult to reach all areas of skin on the body when, just like with dressing the arms, a layer of spongiform fat blocks you from reaching areas that are farther away, like your feet, back, or butt crack. Now, there are workarounds for this too. Just like using a reacher, sock aide, and long-handled shoe horn to aide in lower-body dressing, there are also tools for bathing. The adaptive equipment available for bathing is just as clever—like a long-handled bath brush and handheld shower head. Or there's getting another person to wash the hard-to-reach areas in the darkness for you. "Thanks for saving the best for me, Bob!" says Bob's wife as she washes his out-of-reach body parts. Now that's stoking the fire for you, right?

We have already listed many of the negative health effects of obesity, like increased risk of stroke, diabetes, and death. These detriments are well publicized by our government and schools, yet people still continue to grow larger and move less.

So again, we are turning this up a notch and openly revealing the unknown, secret, personal, and behind-the-scenes reality of obesity and morbid obesity when it comes to a person's quality of life. These topics are not openly talked about or publicized because we are worried about hurting people's feelings, rubbing people the wrong way, or being politically incorrect. Well, how the hell can we fix or heal a problem as big as the current obesity epidemic if we can't even talk about it?

On that note, let's blow the lid off this party can. Let's talk about what's in my opinion, based on my clinical observations and experiences treating thousands of patients over the years in the hospital setting, the worst and most life-altering impairment to self-care that obesity can cause.

The inability to wipe your own ass.

"What the hell! You didn't just go there." Yes, I did.' Cause it's super common. In fact, it's much more common a predicament than anyone realizes. And it's disturbing.

I work with lots of people every day who cannot wipe their own butt. In fact, I would guess that seven out of ten patients who have been admitted to a hospital and *ordered* by their doctors to work with therapists are overweight, obese, or morbidly obese.

Doctors do not order us to see healthy thin, muscular, or skinny people unless they've had surgery or have an unpreventable issue, or if they've ruined their bodies with smoking, drugs, alcohol, or an accident leading to trauma. The low percentage of leaner, lower-weight, active, and healthy people admitted to the hospital are usually there for natural reasons, like baby delivery, broken bones, or some other unpreventable issue.

Basically, healthy people don't need hospitals.

Unhealthy obese patients cannot wipe or poorly wipe after a bowel movement (BM), making a big mess of things due to poor reach ability. They are also eating a lot of greasy, unhealthy food and have multiple BMs a day. Hello, massive, stinky, much-too-frequent, explosive blow-outs.

"Well, how does it get wiped?" you're thinking.

The answer is already there in your mind; you're just blocking it from revealing itself openly because it is so unfathomable, and it's somewhat traumatic for the *non-healthcare worker*:

Another person wipes it.

. . . Or it doesn't get wiped.

This predicament is very sad and much too prevalent in the world. The inability to wipe your own ass after taking a dump is embarrassing and degrading, and it's a complete loss of all dignity or modesty for most people.

The other day I interviewed a gal at a spa in reference to Brazilian bikini waxing for obese clients. "Do you turn people away?" I asked. She replied with a sigh of disgust, "Oh, yeah, you wouldn't believe the stuff we see. We have to tell those people to go home and take care of that first." She was referring to the dirty state of a morbidly obese person's crotch and anus area that gets waxed. In healthcare, this is referred to as the peroneal or peri-area.

There are creative methods for cleaning the peri-area at home that cannot be replicated by an obese person once they have been taken out of their home and placed into a hospital.

Riding a beach towel is a common technique. With one arm grasping the towel in front and the other arm at the back, the person pulls or drags the towel back and forth through the anal-groin area until the crack is clean. Another technique is laying a towel on the edge of the bed or on the towel rack, then rubbing the booty up and down and all around until it is sufficiently cleaned, or as clean as can be expected in this situation. The poopy towel goes in the laundry, or sometimes multiple poopy towels a day if you're a frequent shitter or have diarrhea.

There are many other alternative methods to wipe your butt if you cannot reach it. One option is using a toilet aid. A toilet aid is a long-handled, usually curved, soft plastic and rubber contraption with a catch at the end to wrap toilet paper on. It will extend a person's reach to wipe that booty. Some toilet aids come with a carry case if you're traveling or out on the town. I mean, think about it. If you cannot wipe your butt without your toilet aid, then you definitely don't want to get stuck on a public toilet without it. If there is no beach towel available or sharable wall-mount toilet aid, then you are left with nothing other than pulling up those pants and hoping it doesn't leak through before you make it back home.

Don't worry, if you are obese and this hasn't motivated you enough to start eating restrictively and start an exercise program, there are cool new smart toilets. Smart toilets are high technology. Sitting down initiates a heated seat. After you've pinched off a loaf, the smart toilet will spray a warm-water wash at your butt crack until it is clean as a whistle. To finalize this grand toileting experience, the smart toilet will warm-air blow-dry your buttocks to its splendor.

Not all obese persons are stuck in this exact dilemma, but with different variations, they struggle to wipe that booty. It may not be as easy as when they were thinner, yet if they remain pretty flexible, likely those who are younger than older, they can get the job done using momentum and such.

The poopy-butt dilemma seems to predominantly affect the obese and morbidly obese who are sedentary and deconditioned, retiring, aging, getting sick more often, suffering from urinary tract infections and hygiene-related infections like cellulitis, or starting to need surgeries. They just cannot use flexibility, strength, or momentum to their advantage anymore.

Motivated yet? Well, you should be because this shit is real, and the older you get, the harder it is to backtrack.

EXERLEAN's Butt-Scale and Wipeability Meter was designed to help those visual learners out there. I've developed these simple visual parameters to measure wipeability. There are two basic factors involved in the ability to get a quality reach and wipe. One is the *length of the wiping arm* from shoulder to hand. This length can never change. You cannot separate your shoulder from the body, and your range of motion at the shoulder, elbow, wrist, and hands are fixed and have their limits. The second factor is *butt-cheek size and the open space/width of the butt crack*. The leaner or thinner a person is, the narrower the total butt width from outer hip edge to outer hip edge and the wider, more open the crack or space between the butt cheeks. The lean person with space between their butt cheeks is known as the clean shitter. The poop does not rub on the butt cheeks on the way out, leaving no trace of residue. The fatter the butt, the less open or tighter the butt crack and the wider the butt from outer hip edge to outer hip edge. In other words, the more obese the person, the less space between the cheeks until there is no space at all, like two balloons smashing together and drowning out the butt crack altogether. This is known as the dirty shitter. Poop smears on the cheeks on the way out, leaving much residue for cleanup, which requires more toilet paper, baby wipes, and work.

To get a visual of this scale, imagine sitting on a copy machine and taking a copy of your butt. The more obese the person, the wider the butt printout and also the narrower the butt crack.

EXERLEAN
Butt Scale and Wipeability Meter

Poop Form	Lean/Ripped "The Clean Shitter"	Average "No Problemo"	Overweight "The Struggler"	Obese/Morbidly Obese "Good Luck"
"Deer Poop" Hard Pellet High Protien Diet Bodybuilder	No Residue	Trace Residue	Minimal Wiping	Needs to wipe, big time (can't reach/ use toilet aide)
"Animal" Separates or sticks together Med-High Protien Diet and Fiber	No Residue	Trace Plus+	Moderate Struggle	Needs a Bidet
"The Taper" Human Solid Soft Slider	Trace Wipe	Average Wipe	Difficult Wipe	Bidet + Beach Towel
"The Blow Out" Pressurized loose bowel	Wipe-A-Way	Lots of TP Doable	Shit Everywhere Needs Shower	Impossible Shit Everywhere Needs Shower
"Vomit" out the other end. The Anus Faucet	Multi-wipe Situation	Multi-Wipe+ Bidet	Smeared Bowel Needs Shower + Towel	Apocalypse Needs caregiver assistance

EXERLEAN
Reachability Meter

"As the body widens, the shoulder to hand length remains the same. The further the hand gets from the buttocks, the harder...if not impossible it is to wipe."

No obstruction

Shoulder to hand length

Human body perfecly engineered to reach butt with hand in related position.

Lean / Thin / Light

Shoulder to hand length

Hand to butt distance

Average / Regular / Medium

Body fat becomes obstructive.

Arm length same. Widening torso.

Hand to butt distance increasing. Difficult wipe.

Overweight / Plump / Moderately Heavy

Width of torso and buttocks decreases reachability

Cannot reach. Impossible to wipe.

Obese / Morbidly Obese / Super Heavy

Adaptive methods and equipment can help a person wipe when they cannot reach the poop. For example, a toilet aide, an over-tiolet bidet, or smart toilet. The best remedy is to lose weight.

Now is your time to act. Remember! The current way of thinking, and the trends and statistics we have reviewed so far, are bad and in a sharp upward climb to oblivion.

The Obesiboomer generation is paying a high price and will continue to pay more physically, mentally, financially, and with decreased overall quality of life. As the prevalence of obesity continues to rise, so will the Obesiboomers' decline in occupational performance, community mobility, and self-care.

The well-publicized health detriments listed by the CDC, the World Health Organization (WHO), and the NIH will continue to skyrocket out of control.

The current education system in schools, in public health sectors, and on social media about the negative effects of obesity and how to deal with them is *obviously* not working!

In fact, the current social and education environment is teaching us that in a way, obesity is a "good thing" and should be accepted. Social media outlets and news broadcasts have been force-feeding us information and reeducation, brainwashing us into believing that being overweight, obese, and morbidly obese is beautiful, normal, and to be considered such.

Hate to break it to you—this is a nontruth.

A lie.

This kind of media and force-fed education is teaching our youth, average adults, and the general public that being overweight, obese, and morbidly obese should be considered normal and to accept it as such.. . . Bullshit!

Don't succumb to this ruse.

No wonder the obesity epidemic is afflicting so many youth, adults, and the elderly at rates exponentially increasing as every year passes. No wonder we as a species are becoming fatter and fatter year by year.

We need to change our way of thinking and our view on being overweight, obese, and morbidly obese.

We need to stay focused on the truth. The truth that excess body fat is a predictor of negative health consequences, and the more obese a person is, the worse the afflictions they will face, leading all the way to and possibly causing death.

This is the primary driver for me writing this book. I see what is happening in the hospitals, in schools, and in public, and I monitor the statistics on obesity. Nothing out there is working to halt the rising statistics on child, adult, and elderly obesity, and death is on the horizon. Nothing the government, schools, and medical community are doing is decreasing the rise in the obesity epidemic.

That is why I am approaching this problem at such a different angle.

I want to make a positive difference in people's lives and bring about a trend that will hopefully end the obesity epidemic—otherwise referred to as the Obesiboomer epidemic or pandemic, you might say. My goal is to give you enough ammunition. Enough reason to treat and prevent obesity now and for the rest of your life.

The Obesiboomer epidemic is spreading like wildfire, and the knowledge of health detriments like diabetes, stroke, heart attack, and death do not seem to be giving people enough ammunition or motivation to do the work, to make positive changes toward their health.

Hopefully, getting a glimpse into how being overweight, obese, or morbidly obese can affect the unseen, intimate, private, and very personal aspects of your life is enough knowledge, enough fuel, to explode that motivation train into full steam ahead. The negative side effects and reality of obesity we discuss openly in this book are meant to slap you across the face to get your attention, then reach inside you, grab your soul, and shake it around a bit. The goal is to help you retain this knowledge with the hope that it sticks in the back of your mind forever. You may not be ready to do something about your body fat now, but maybe down the road something from this book will click, and EXERLEAN will be waiting. I want you to think about all the devastating effects of obesity every time you are about to sink your teeth into something to eat. When you are eating, I want you to think about what specifically you are eating and whether it is necessary energy, whether it is healthy, and whether it will go toward healing your body or get sent straight to your ass to get stored there!

That, I hope, will help motivate you to do what is necessary now and for the rest of your life. To lose all the excess body fat and start exercising.

This is EXERLEAN: restrictive + healthy + balanced nutrition, daily exercise, and hyperactive activities of daily living. It's the formula for achieving happiness, longevity, and living without difficulty.

Daily exercise plus healthy and restrictive nutrition . . . you cannot have one without the other.

you + EXERLEAN = maximal health

EXERcising daily + eating LEAN
EXER + LEAN = EXERLEAN

If all Obesiboomers follow and live by the EXERLEAN formula, there will eventually be no more Obesiboomers. The perfect scenario would be a shift of the obesity statistics in a different direction. A new era of humanity focused on their health management, working toward maintaining a healthy body weight and staying active with work, play, and exercise. Maybe this book will help create an army of health nuts, fitness gurus, health and wellness coaches, bodybuilders, CrossFitters, power-lifters, gymnasts, dancers, martial artists, runners, bicyclers, hikers, and other physically active people. The dawn of the Leanbodiboomers.

You're reading this book because you want change. You want to do something different from the norm. Something that will help you down the path to looking better, feeling better, having more energy, being stronger, sleeping better, elevating your sex and libido, and living a longer and rewarding healthstyle.

Good! That is why I wrote this book, and trust me, it will help you make radical changes to the way you look at life, yourself, and the human body, and how to remediate and/or prevent the health detriments of obesity in your life.

Please don't skip ahead.

The information in the book from beginning to end is strategically laid out to help you transform yourself into the *best you ever*. I want you to fully grasp why this works and why you are doing what you are going to be doing. This information will help you for the rest of your life. Learn the rules, principles, and process, then you can achieve a life living lean forever. Some of the materials are designed with the intent to provoke you, to wake up your inner passion, and to help reboot your healthstyle, which will help you achieve a *real* transformation.

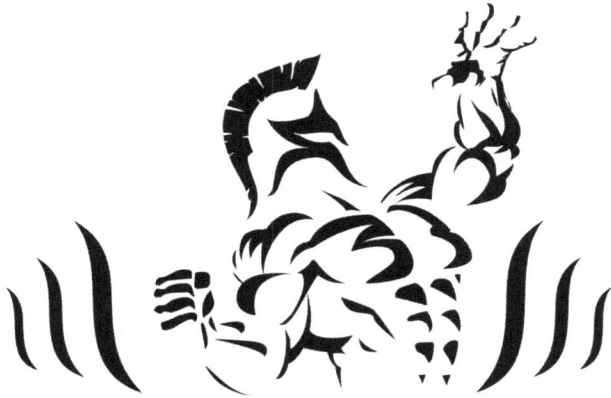

TOTAL BODY FAT
INCINERATOR

TOTAL BODY FAT
INCINERATOR

CONTENTS

CHAPTER 9
HIGH BIOLOGICAL VALUE PROTEINS

We already discussed nitro—when your blood is chock-full of amino acids—and how a continuous supply of protein to your bloodstream helps maintain a positive nitrogen state in your body. A positive nitrogen state is when your body retains more nitrogen than it puts out—nitrogen in versus nitrogen out. When your body is more nitrogen in than out, you are in an anabolic state, where lean mass preservation is at its best, especially when you're on a restrictive diet or in an energy-deprived state. Continuously supplying your body with proteins promotes healing, growth, and prevention of muscle cannibalism. Positive nitrogen or nitro blood is key, and high biological protein is king.

The body values amino acids, unlike carbohydrates or fats. Remember, amino acids are the only nutrition our bodies can use to heal damaged cells, heal wounds, and recover from work. Carbohydrates and fats cannot heal the body. In fact, carbohydrate-saturated blood, or sweet blood, leads to diabetes and all its negative outcomes like poor circulation, low vision, poor wound healing, and tissue death. Fat-laden blood, or sludge blood, leads to plaque buildup and crystallization of the arterial wall, putting you at high risk of stroke, heart attack, and death.

Therefore, preventing sweet blood or sludge blood and maintaining nitro is vital in achieving a state of health and wellness.

The proteins you feed your body to attain a positive nitrogen state are not all created equal. Just as there are many grades of fuel that deliver varying levels of performance, protein comes in many grades of quality. The higher quality the protein, the better performance of your body. For example, diesel obviously delivers less performance than rocket fuel, and low biological value protein delivers less performance than high biological protein. In your quest to achieve your physical best, you want to feed your body with the best proteins possible, proteins with high biologic value, just as an Indy 500 racer wants the highest performance fuel attainable so they may win the race.

The biological value (BV) scale is a protein rating scale from 0 to 100. The higher the BV rating, the better the quality of protein. A protein source that has a score of 100 percent is completely utilized for growth, healing, and maintaining lean body mass. The higher the protein BV rating, the better *usability* factor. The lower the BV rating, the less likely the protein food source will be used by your body for protein-related physiology.

Whey protein and eggs are two top-tier, high BV proteins. Most if not all animal-based proteins have a high biological value for the purposes of protein—namely, to supply amino acids for materializing new muscle tissue, healing, and revitalization. Low-BV protein sources have less usability for protein's purposes.

Digesting and then assimilating food sources refers to the natural occurrence of breaking down a food source into its constituents— proteins, carbs, and fats. You can focus on the purpose of carbohydrates or the purpose of fats, but the BV scale looks specifically at the quality of a protein and the body's ability to use it for the purposes of protein.

Some protein sources on the BV scale, especially those rated lower, have value for the purposes of protein and value for the purposes of carbohydrates and/or fats. All protein sources provide calories, but the calories may be from something other than protein, as in the case of soy. Soybeans are rated on the BV scale, yet they are a carbohydrate source by nature. Much of the calorie content of soybeans is provided in the form of glucose. You will have to eat much more soybeans to achieve the quantity of protein per grams necessary compared to true protein sources, like meat, fish, eggs, and whey. Protein sources on the BV scale, like soy protein, are less "usable" for the body compared to protein sources higher on the BV scale.

Animal-based protein sources are high biological value protein, yet depending on the cut of meat, they may be used for the purposes of protein *and* the purposes of fat. In your EXERLEAN protocol, fat consumption is minimized to encourage body fat burning, not storage. Therefore, your mission is to choose lean high-biological-value protein sources that contribute to the purposes of protein, not fat.

Most people look at food labels to figure out the ratio, usually in grams, of protein, carbohydrates, and fat. Now that you know every protein is not created equal, you can make sure you are buying and consuming high biological value protein. High BV protein that your body will use for the purposes of protein and not for energy.

When you are looking at any food label, you should not count up the grams of protein in carbohydrate foods like a loaf of bread. A slice of bread might list 4 grams of protein, but this is low biological value, low usability for your body for the purposes of protein. If you ate the whole loaf of bread, say twenty slices, you would benefit from 80 grams of low biological value protein and 2,400-plus calories of mostly energy, which if not burned off in active work would go straight to body fat.

Obviously eating an entire loaf of bread at once is totally unrealistic and unhealthy, but the concept is the same if you were to eat it over a week's time.

Only count protein grams from high BV protein sources. Do not add in low-BV protein sources to your daily protein count. Low BV protein that comes from things like bread, donuts, crackers, rice, and oats are not quality or sufficient sources of protein for healing, muscle synthesis, and rejuvenation.

Keep carbohydrate sources what they are—energy content. Keep fats what they are—lipids, cholesterol, and fatty acids. Protein is king, and high biological value is a must for your total body fat incineration.

CHAPTER 10
GLYCOGEN DEPLETION

The key tool in the EXERLEAN Diet protocol is harnessing the power of the State, your total body fat incinerator. This maximal force of fat-burning potential lies deep within your body, just waiting to be ignited.

In the world of bodybuilding, when we start talking about glycogen depletion, you know things are heating up, as in fat-burning furnace coming soon! It's a simple concept; take away the body's fuel, and it will resort to the fuel stored in its fat ass, thunder thighs, batwings, double chin, chubby cheeks, beer gut, tummy tires, and cankles. Damn! Ridding your body of all that excess body fat is going to feel so good!

So far, we have reviewed some vital aspects of nutrition most people are unaware of, from the quality of a protein and how usable it is based on a *biological value* rating to the *glycemic rating* of a carbohydrate and the resulting blood sugar and insulin response. We have discussed the benefits of *fasting* and *loading* macronutrients to achieve key results in our dieting endeavors as well as busting through or preventing a plateau in our physical transformation. You are now well aware of the enemy, *sweet blood*, the root cause of obesity, and how to prevent it at all times by maintaining a high-content, high BV protein and low-quantity, low-GI-carbohydrate diet. *Hunger* is a well-established demon in the journey you are about to begin, and only high willpower, discipline, and self-drive can defeat this enemy. You have the fortitude to do this and will!

You have the benefits of EXERLEAN at your side, the combination of exercise and eating lean. You cannot have one without the other and be successful long term. You are preparing to lean yourself out of all the heavy-handed negative choices in life. You are ready to fulfill your lean body destiny by making only the heavy-handed beneficial decisions, leading to a life of the least possible regret.

Future you is on the horizon, and you do not want it to be a future of obesity, morbid obesity, or sarcopenia. Body fat only leads to sickness, disease, disability, poorer quality of life, and high death risk.

Not you, oh, definitely not you. Your future is going to be walking around in a lightweight, lean, strong, and healthy body.

Likely the most important and vital skill for you to harness to achieve the State of fat burning, your total body fat incinerator, is glycogen depletion.

When obesity has taken hold of your body, a reset is necessary. Nothing will shock your body more than depleting all your muscle and liver glycogen, or stored complex carbohydrates. To recap, 5–6 percent of your liver's weight and 1–2 percent of all your muscle weight is glycogen. Your body contains approximately 600 grams of glycogen. The more lean muscle mass you have, the more glycogen you will store. Each gram of glycogen binds with 4 to 5 grams of water, accounting for 2,400 to 3,000 grams of total glycogen weight, which is 5.29 to 6.61 pounds of body weight coming from glycogen alone. When you lower your caloric intake to lose weight, your body will access its glycogen stores for energy if necessary.

If your daily diet includes carbohydrates regardless of calorie intake, your body will continue to replenish and pull from glycogen as needed to maintain your body's set points. When you are consuming a carbohydrate diet, it is nearly impossible to achieve a true state of glycogen depletion. The fastest way to achieve total glycogen depletion is through fasting from carbohydrates. When you don't eat carbs, your body cannot replenish lost glycogen and will pull from glycogen to maintain blood sugar and provide energy for life until all 5 to 7 pounds of your body's glycogen stores are fully depleted. At that point, ketosis sets in.

Ketosis occurs when your body has no carbohydrates to convert to glucose, and all glycogen stores are empty. In this state, your body will go catabolic. Remember, catabolism is cannibalism of your body through internal metabolic processes. Without glucose to use for energy, your body will start pulling from body fat storage—adipose tissue—to use for energy. Your body can also break down lean muscle tissue for energy and processes requiring amino acids.

I have made it clear that the breakdown of lean muscle tissue is the worst result that can occur in a dieting regimen. The loss of lean body tissue, or muscle mass, lowers your metabolic rate, leading to less calorie-burning potential—i.e., less fat burning. The more muscle mass your body has, the more calories it needs for life; therefore, the more fat-burning potential.

When your body enters a ketosis state, it will mostly burn off body fat, not muscle. But to prevent the breakdown of any lean body mass, there are a couple of things you can do: maintain a positive nitrogen state through consistent high BV protein loading and heavy weight training. While strict dieting, heavy weight training will trick your body into holding on to lean body mass purely out of necessity, because with consistent heavy work, your body knows it needs the muscle to do the work and will therefore prioritize body fat metabolism. We will be discussing these topics in upcoming chapters, so for now, let's talk a little more about ketosis.

Ketosis is the basis of all ketogenic diets. This is because there is no more powerful way to burn off body fat than preventing glucose use for fuel. But this is where the EXERLEAN Diet changes things up. The EXERLEAN Diet uses the power of the State, an algorithm for fat burning that harnesses the benefits of fat burning during the process of reaching—but not maintaining—ketosis. In the State, your body hovers just out of ketosis, benefiting from a glycogen-deprived state yet avoiding the negative side effects of the ketosis state.

As we said in an earlier chapter, in any ketogenic diet, the basic idea is fasting from carbs and eating a high-protein, high-fat diet. Fat becomes the fuel replacement for carbohydrates. So, then, how much fat consumption is necessary? How much fat consumption leads to cardiac, arterial, or venous disease? How much fat will kill your possibility at longevity? This is an unknown. Every person has a different metabolism. Every person has different genetics and inherited traits. A lean person can eat fat and has a better chance of staying healthy than an obese person, who has a higher tendency to attain disease from eating fat.

Fat on lean is energy.

Fat on fat is more fat. Sludge blood.

Ketosis is a natural physiologic process the body goes through in a fasting state, when it's deprived of glucose for fuel and insulin that signals to the body, "Hey, blood sugar is coming, get ready to suck it up."

No glucose, no insulin, and your body resorts to body fat to take glucose's job. Body fat is broken down into fatty acids and delivered to your bloodstream. Your liver converts fatty acids to *ketone bodies*, which are delivered to your brain and body for fuel. There is a much more com-plicated explanation for the process of ketosis and the resulting ketone bodies, but it is unnecessary to get super scientific here. All that matters in the end is that when you eat carbs, they supply your body with energy for work. When your body is starved of carbohydrates and your glycogen stores are depleted, your body goes into a state of ketosis, in which body fat is broken down and replaces glucose as energy for work.

The human body is masterfully efficient. The machine is perfectly designed to maintain life in times of desperation, famine, starvation, and other natural phenomena. Your body is always preparing to survive.

Your body is designed to store excess calories as body fat. At times of calorie starvation, body fat is ready and waiting as a dense, high-energy fuel source. Too bad most of us no longer need body fat for survival.

Here's something to think about. If all the excess food that is converted to body fat in at least 72 percent of overweight and obese humans was not eaten and instead send to the areas of the earth dealing with famine, we would likely be able to cure the condition of famine. It is an uneven distribution of food, and I challenge you to eat only what your body needs to be healthy, strong, and immune to disease and disorder (more on that in my book *Pandemic Armor*).

Gluttony is the excessive overconsumption of food, drink, material luxuries, and nowadays, the internet and high technology. To be a glutton is not a good thing. In some religions, gluttony is considered sinful. Overeating and the placard of obesity is a state of reckless abandon. People eat themselves into an unhealthy, diseased, and eventually disabled state by living without considering the consequences of their actions. All the while, others starve in an environment without food, adequate shelter, and technology.

Starving yourself of a macronutrient while at the same time having abundant food around is a lucky state to be in, so count your lucky stars. By cutting out carbohydrates and fat, you will not die. You will thrive. Your body is sick and tired of the gluttony. Sick and tired of the sedentary behavior. Begging you to stop overeating the hyperpalatable shit foods that are bogging you down.

Glycogen depletion is the precursor to ketosis. Ketosis is the precursor to breaking down body fat for fuel. Glycogen depletion occurs through carbohydrate depletion. Stop eating carbs . . . burn off body fat.

To harness the fat-burning potential of ketosis and spare lean body mass simultaneously requires maintaining a positive nitrogen state within your body.

CHAPTER 11
POSITIVE NITROGEN

We have touched on nitrogen in the body and the benefits of maintaining a positive nitrogen state, but why? The opposite is a negative nitrogen state. A negative nitrogen environment in the body is a catastrophic outcome of famine, fasting, or dieting done wrong. The nitrogen in your body can be positive, negative, or teetering in and out of equilibrium. Negative nitrogen balance must be avoided at all times, at all costs, for your entire life. The catabolic or cannibalistic results of being in a negative nitrogen state for the long term are muscle wasting, decreased immunity, decreased overall work output, and possible sarcopenia.

Nitrogen promotes good things in your body. This is because nitrogen is directly related to protein intake, and protein itself is the building block of all things physical in your body. All healing requires protein. All rejuvenation requires protein. Immunity is bolstered by having a solid core of lean body mass. Metabolic rate is directly related to the presence and quantity of lean muscle tissue. The more muscle on your body, the better your immune system, the higher your metabolic rate, the better your work productivity, and the higher the workload you can muster. Your brain and muscles do the work, so your brain and muscles use the bulk of all consumed energy.

The amount of nitrogen in your body is a good predictor of your health, your ability to prevent lean muscle cannibalism, and your potential for physical recovery. Your blood is the vital aspect of your body's physiology, and what it carries will predict your body composition and your disease or health status. As you know, blood carries all nutrients you consume—fat, carbohydrates, and protein—breaking them down and then absorbing and transporting them to wherever they are needed. If unneeded, they will be expelled from your body or stored for later use.

You ultimately choose the foods that go in your mouth; therefore, you are the master and commander of your blood chemistry. Eat high fat, enjoy the negative consequences that sludge blood gifts you. Eat high carbohydrates, be rewarded with potent energy and a sweet-blood watershed of metabolic chaos that leads to obesity and disease. Consume high amounts of protein, and enjoy the benefits of being in a positive nitrogen state, feeling the power of maximal lean body mass and the benefits of anabolism.

Take comfort by knowing your body is at a higher probability of being nitrogen positive by consuming a diet of high BV proteins. High BV proteins loaded at a consistent rate and timed strategically to maximize anabolism, along with body fat thermogenesis, is vital to attaining and maintaining a positive nitrogen environment. A positive nitrogen state is a prerequisite of the EXERLEAN Diet and key in achieving the State of ultimate body fat incineration.

In the State, your body will be energy deprived, forcing you to replace lost energy with body fat.

In the State, your body will be nitrogen positive, ensuring that while you're incinerating body fat, you are also *not* incinerating lean body mass.

In the State, you will stimulate your body with weightlifting, which will help maintain at a minimum or improve your lean body core.

In the State, you will use fasting and carbohydrate loading to harness the power of shocking your body, keeping it guessing to prevent accommodation or a plateau.

In the State, you will prevent sweet blood at all costs.

In the State, you will prevent sludge blood at all costs.

In the State, you will harness the thermogenic power of ketosis yet not be in ketosis, preventing ketone bodies from spilling.

In the State, you will be following a scientifically strategic protocol to control your body. Your body will do what you want it to do—incinerate body fat, prevent reaccumulation of body fat, and maximize lean body structures.

Positive nitrogen equals positive gains.

CHAPTER 12
PROTEIN LOADING

In the world of fad diets, celebrity diets, and seasonal diets, you hear about carbohydrate loading and in the ketogenic diet about fat loading, but you don't hear much about protein loading. Why is this?

Fear.

Avoidance.

Fear of the unknown? Unwarranted fear of what? Animal right activists? The strict vegan who may view eating animal products as a sin or inherently wrong? Lack of research? Kidney failure? Why do we dance around the topic of protein loading? Who knows!

If we are willing to accept that the ketogenic diet and high-fat consumption is okay at the risk of coronary artery disease, or that a diet high in carbohydrates is okay at the risk of adult-onset diabetes, then why do we not explore openly the idea that eating primarily protein may be okay?

We develop the preconceived biases in our psyche through modeling, learning, and experience. We grow up with the idea that the "full-course meal" is a prerequisite to your personal health and wellness . . . and don't forget dessert! Talk about a big dose of extra body fat. The full-course meal is okay once in a while, but it is not conducive to maintaining a lean body.

The human body only needs the nutrients it needs at the time, and protein is always needed. Work requires an energy expenditure; therefore, calories are needed. When in a resting state, the body only needs to satisfy the resting metabolic rate, which can be done with body fat alone. In fact, burning off body fat in a resting state may be the preferred path of body fat incineration. If you're also in a positive nitrogen state and devoid of energy calories, a resting state will spare your lean body mass in preference of adipose tissue. In the EXERLEAN protocol, this is referred to as *fasted sleep* or *fasted rest.*

So long as you are protein loading, that is, providing your body with a steady stream of high biological value protein, your body's potential for a positive nitrogen state is maximized—and while you're sleeping, you may burn off body fat, simultaneously healing and rejuvenating your body from the day's workload trauma. It is a wild idea, but one that highly experienced bodybuilding and fitness competitors use on a routine basis. The science of this is not well researched, but the pragmatic and objective results seen in everyday life of bodybuilders is enough justification to give it a try.

What do you have to lose?

Body fat, that's what!

Protein loading can take many different formats, and every person has a different experience. You will need to monitor your body composition, journal your progress, and modify your nutritional intake as necessary throughout your transformation. One person may need to consume protein every two hours, another every four hours. An active person may need around 40 grams of protein every two hours, whereas a heavy but lean muscular person may need 80 grams every three hours. It all depends on the person's amount of lean body mass, time in labor, time under tension or physical stress, calorie expenditure, and metabolic rate.

Just like fasting for a day can jolt the system and achieve great results to rest the body, burn body fat, and clean out your blood, eating only protein for a day induces the nitrogen state, leans out glucose, and primes you for a thermogenic response.

Fibrous Vegetable Loading

Another invaluable complement to protein loading is adding in a truckload of fibrous low-calorie vegetables. Fibrous vegetable loading is key to satiety in a complex-carbohydrate-restricted state and, for most of the EXERLEAN protocol, to maintain the State of total body fat incineration.

Fibrous vegetables are very low in calories, and some are actually negative calorie value as they take more calories to digest and assimilate than is present in them. They add the benefit of volume, triggering the vagal reflex (bowel distention), and help you reach a state of satiety and satisfaction. Fibrous vegetable loading is likely your best weapon against the evil obesity conjurer, hunger.

Fibrous vegetable loading with protein loading also helps you digest and assimilate protein better than without fiber. That's because foods rich in fiber help move food through the intestines. Protein in the form of meat is more difficult and takes longer for the body to break down, digest, and assimilate than carbohydrates and fats. Fibrous vegetables are more difficult for the body to break down compared to starchy complex and simple carbohydrates. Any slowing or extending of the digestion process is beneficial as it decreases the chance of overwhelming the system with calories, thus helping to prevent storing more body fat.

PART 2

ENTER

The Total Body Fat Incinerator

It is finally your time.

Harnessing the power of the State, the EXERLEAN total body fat incinerator is a strategic and disciplined physiologic process that will help you earn your lean, hard body. Everything until now delivered the foundational information you need to know and retain in order to successfully go through the self-discovery process of your body, your metabolism, and your psychological, mental, and spiritual self.

The negative consequences of the mere state of being overweight or obese are well founded, researched, and documented. There is no doubt whatsoever that excessive body fat is an unwelcome burden. Obesity is a life sentence of variable degrees of disease, disability, poor quality of life, and possible onset of early mortality. Just as a criminal deserves their charges, so does the obese person earn their health consequences, as crime and excessive body fat are both 100 percent preventable. Both reap the benefits of the most regret.

Excessive body fat is unnecessary in this life. The technological advancements of our civilization have surmounted the survival necessities of our ancestors. Any debate that body fat is necessary to keep us warm and provide energy during famine is a dead-end conversation that ended in the early 1900s.

The Obesiboomer movement is exponentially climbing toward total human fatness. If the onset of obesity does not stop, the majority of the earth will be obese sooner than imagined. It's frickin' disgusting if you really think about it. The lack of willpower, the reckless abandon for our health, the life of regret we accept, the state of excessive body fat most of us disregard.

No more shall we accept this *fat* ass shit!

No more shall we live in regret and with wishful thinking.

You are going to take action *now*, before it is too late and the negative effects of obesity take you out.

The process to burn off body fat is easy when you execute the action steps correctly and maintain discipline to the algorithm. The state of body fat thermogenesis is at hand. You need only to unlock the code to turn on your total body fat incinerator.

CHAPTER 13
THE STATE

I am excited to introduce you to the nucleus of the deal, the algorithm to unlock your total body fat incinerator. There is nothing more rewarding for me to see than people positively changing their lives by making healthy choices followed by the necessary action steps to achieve personal renewal. I am proud you have come this far, and I believe in you. Everything you have learned up to this point has built the foundation for success in what you are going to do next—dieting. Getting lean should be everyone's health goal, to improve present and future quality of life, maintain independence with self-care, and thrive in a productive society. With obesity, the negative rewards are heavy handed. You must burn off all the body fat.

You can do this.

I don't need to tell you that dieting is a rough road. What I can tell you is that the results of executing this algorithm will be worth the work.

Imagine your thin skin, improved muscle tone, less weight on your feet, and being able to see your nether regions and your feet. You're going to get so lean, wiping your ass will never be difficult again. Your rolls of belly fat will have been incinerated, and now you can slide your hands down your belly, rolling over each washboard ridge as though you're handwashing your laundry. Imagine your inner thighs with a space between them. No more thick fat legs chaffing together with every step you take. No more shopping for fat-ass jeans. Tight and toned is your new mantra. When people lay their eyes on you, health is obvious, and inspiration transpires. Be ready to be followed.

"Let's do this!"

Your Diet?

diet: *food and drink regularly provided or consumed; habitual nourishment; the kind and amount of food prescribed for a person or animal for a special reason; a regimen of eating and drinking sparingly so as to reduce one's weight; something provided or experienced repeatedly (Merriam-Webster)*

EXERLEAN takes only what works for dieting and incorporates it into the program. Anything that doesn't work or has lackluster results has been eliminated to save you time. The EXERLEAN Diet combines the best methods of fat burning and the best formulas for lean mass preservation to help you design a routine diet that will lead you to maximal health. EXERLEAN incorporates many aspects of the dieting protocols competitive bodybuilders use to achieve atypical, extraordinary results.

Your time is valuable and nonrefundable. We must make every minute count toward positive, productive, and rewarding outcomes.

You need to understand that no one specific method or diet will work for the long term. The best long-term results come from a program that uses different methods of varying, cycling, fasting, and refeeding. This is because the body will adapt to any specific method after a prolonged time. Variation prevents adaption and promotes continued changes in your body, which will help you prevent or bust out of a plateau.

EXERLEAN: *The State* is a dieting algorithm designed to keep your body guessing and changing for the better, to prevent plateaus, and to help you maintain the results of your hard work for the long term.

When the State has been achieved, the body is forced to devour its own body fat through the metabolic pathway. The State algorithm unlocks your internal total body fat incinerator. Achieving the State of ultimate body fat incineration takes a disciplined and focused approach. All the steps and criteria must be met for a successful outcome; do not derail, cheat, or sabotage your mission. It is complicated science, but I've simplified it in this book.

The State of ultimate body fat incineration is a three-stage algorithm that's two weeks long and easy to follow. Easy, yes, but discipline and mental fortitude will be paramount for your success.

Burn this in your brain: the best things in life are not easy to garner but are forged in time by your inner blacksmith.

Ultimately, you make you. Your body is the result of your eating choices and activity level over the course of time. The environment you live in, your daily routine, and the people who surround you are the results of choices you have made. You put yourself where you are at any given moment. You weren't forced into this position! The people and environment you've chosen will attempt to influence you—to coerce you to maintain the status quo. Even coworkers and family fight change within the group. They do not appreciate an outlier, who makes the standbys feel uncomfortable and possibly inadequate. Only you can make choices based on the triggers around you.

Are you unhappy?

Change is necessary.

Seek at all times to be the outlier.

Envision your future self, and do the work necessary to make future you a reality. This is just a guide to help you get there faster. Many of the skills in discipline and mental fortitude you will learn during this fat-burning process can be used in many other ambitions in your life. Arnold Schwarzenegger knew this. He took the same discipline, work ethic, and confidence that bodybuilding built in him and put it toward his other ambitions of acting, politics, and social influence. Arnold is an outlier.

"I can do this with or without you, naysayers!" says future you.

Now, let's get down to business!

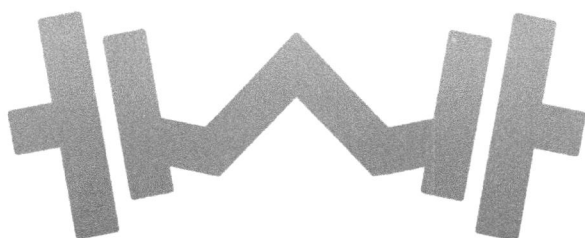

TEASER 3

WEIGHT CHAINING

CONTENTS

TRAILER

You have returned to planet earth and cannot believe what you see. Fat humans . . . skinny-fat, potbellied, apple and pear shaped, and many other odd distortions of the human anatomy. Obesity and weakness are of epidemic status. We have evolved into a corpulent human race.

"My, lord," you say to yourself. In disbelief and astonishment, you gawk.

It is a mind-blowing sight, from that of a long-gone member of society such as yourself. Welcome back from Mars! Welcome home.

The majority of human beings are now overweight, obese, or super-morbidly obese. Most are working less, are weaker, are sedentary, and have wrecked their fat-burning metabolisms. Technology has surpassed manual labor, putting the human body out of work. Computers, AI, and robotics are taking over the show. Humans need only think, plan, and press buttons to control all things around them. Amazon . . . anything! Fast food . . . dine-in, takeout, or delivery. Groceries . . . delivered. Manual labor jobs are becoming scarce; jobs filled with maximal sit time have replaced them. Automobiles, planes, e-bikes, hoverboards, power scooters, subways, and trains have replaced manual locomotion. Power recliners, lift chairs, power adjustable beds, escalators, automatic doors, elevators, power scooters, and power shopping carts have replaced the work of the lower extremities. Many humans lack the labor, workload, exercise, and weight-bearing activity necessary for the body to survive and thrive.

Welcome to the age of obesity, sarcopenia, sarcopenic obesity, weakness, and failure to thrive. Obesity and sedentary behavior are taking a huge toll on the majority of people . . . a death toll. Quality of life and self-care function are greatly diminished for many of these hefty humans. Typically, the older a hefty human gets, the worse they feel and the less they function. The earth's gravity, or resistance, is also taking an exponential toll on people's body structures. Obesity increases mass on top of the already persistent resistant forces of gravity. The negative effects of being obese in a gravity environment compound like a stack of pancakes.

The last time you visited earth was over a century ago, and oh, how things have changed. The technological advancements are impressive for sure. No more walking to work, as most own an automobile, use a public transit system, or rideshare. Sedentary behavior is the name of the beast, and it has overcome humanity. The productivity of a worker is less than halved. In the home, people enjoy AI- and Wi-Fi–enabled wells pumps, dishwashers, laundry machines, remote controls, robotic vacuums, hot water tanks, and air conditioning. Twenty-four-hour-a-day clean water is available at the tap, and an abundance of food sits in refrigerators and freezers. Most everything has been automated and workloads reduced or eliminated. Television and smartphones are the new fixes.

Not only have people gotten bigger, but so have their houses. There are millions of houses scattered across the country that would have been considered mansions in the last century. What is considered a mansion now would have been considered a castle a century ago. Big houses need more work to keep them healthy and clean, but homeowners aren't the ones doing much of the work. Housekeeping, pool cleaning, lawn care, and other services are prominently used to care for these big homes . . . just like big people require care to keep them clean and functional. No one has to lift a finger anymore. Unless people supplement their sedentary lives with exercise, weight training, and recreational activity, they are at high risk of being doomed to an unfulfilling life and possibly death before their time. This is because the muscles and bony structure of the body need the resistance of a workload, the same as the body needs oxygen to breathe or water to drink.

Manual labor is scarce.

Food is abundant.

Work has transformed to that of the mind and mouth and less of the brawn.

Muscles are poorly toned and shrinking.

Body fat sacks are overflowing as sedentary behavior and food over-consumption prevail.

Welcome to the dawn of the Obesiboomers.

According to the 2013–2014 National Health and Nutrition Examination Survey (NHANES), more than one in three adults are overweight, two out of three adults are overweight or obese, and one out of six children are obese.

The overall consensus is that 70-plus percent of people in the US are at a minimum overweight, and likely obese or teetering on the edge of obesity.

Much research has been done on the sedentary behavior of "sit time," which encompasses screen time, workplace sitting, time in a car seat, and sitting at home, and links it to compromised metabolic health and early mortality . . . that is, death sooner than later.

Can you say *obese sedentary death*?

Not a good way to go.

INTRODUCTION

Y ou would think that with the advancements in technology, research, and science that things would have gone the other way for the human race. Knowledge on human physiology, metabolism, exercise, and food are well known. Unless you have been living in a Wi-Fi–free cave in a third-world country, you are aware that overeating leads to fatness and that sedentary behavior leads to muscle atrophy, slower metabolism, and weakness. These consequences are well documented and widely taught.

This should be the dawn of the lean and healthy humans, not this fat and indolent shitstorm.

What the heck is happening here on planet earth?

Let's begin the journey to your lean and muscular body, your lighter and faster body, your maximal self-confidence and personal satisfaction with your body by first unraveling the truth. Only then can we unseat the problem, discover the path to success, and prepare you for a physical transformation.

The indolent shitstorm?

Who is to blame?

Well, the reality is . . .

You are to blame. It is your fault that you are lean, healthy, strong, fat, unhealthy, or weak. You control you. Nobody else can make you eat too much, drink too little, do drugs, drink protein shakes, smoke anything, take vitamins, eat vegetables and meat, liposuck your face to look slimmer, run on a treadmill, or binge-watch TV while lying back in a recliner.

Go ahead . . . throw this book at the wall. It won't do you any good, though. If you are out of shape and unhealthy, that is the same reaction that has led you to being overweight or obese, atrophied, weak, and unfulfilled. It is the reaction of deflection. The "not me" mentality. It is much easier to blame, justify, and complain than it is to accept responsibility for one's own situation, especially when it comes to body composition.

But you are likely reading this book because you want to change, right?

Good. Change is necessary.

Your need to transform your body, healthstyle, and nutritional profile is vital for your survival.

Your present and future depend on what you do now . . . before it's too late and obesity, aging, and sedentary weakness incapacitate you.

There is hope.

All the badness is caused by choices we make. Because the choices we make are exactly that—a choice between what we decide or what we could have decided. There must be an alternate pathway that doesn't lead to the shitstorm. There must have been a good pathway we dismissed. This means that all the badness is preventable.

It's not the fault of the choice but that of the decision-makers.

Awareness of the negative effects of sedentary behavior, poor nutrition, and being out of shape or obese is the first step toward change. You can then acknowledge the negative effects of unhealthy behaviors on the body and use this information as fuel for transformation—to find treatment. If these consequences aren't fuel, they should be, 'cause the shit that people, especially the aging, deal with when they have lived a life of overindulgence, gluttony, and sedentary behavior is devastating. The badness just adds up . . . bad choice after bad after bad. The negative effects of having low muscle bulk, low tone, unnecessary body fat, weakness, poor metabolism, and the diseases and disabilities that come with it all turn out to be the ingredients for regret.

Sarcopenia is a loss of muscle mass and with it, loss of brute strength and power, which then negatively affects your ability to engage in activities of daily living and functional mobility. Another way to describe sarcopenia is muscle wasting. This is usually the result of cumulative sedentary behavior, absence of exercise, absence of weightlifting, insufficient protein consumption, and aging.

Sarcopenia, low muscle mass, and the frailty associated with it can be used to predict a person's detriment and discharge location from a hospital. People lacking adequate muscle are weaker, are less resilient, have less reserve energy to sustain work, and are more likely to be placed in a destination other than their home when they're discharged—for example, to a rehab center, assisted living facility, or nursing home.

Every choice we make from childhood to teen, young adult, middle age, and pre-retirement lays the foundation for whether your golden years will be exactly that—golden, or crappy brown and full of pain, despair, and regret.

I can attest to this negative outcome as an occupational therapist (OT) and a Certified Aging-in-Place Specialist (CAPS). Most hospital therapists, nurses, and doctors adopt a skewed view of humanity after spending most of our week at work where the majority of admitted patients have chronic sickness, disease, disabling medical issues, and other unpleasant situations that prevent them from thriving. After forty to fifty hours a week working in the hospital, year after year, seeing only the bad, how could anyone not adopt a negative view of what aging and retirement really mean? If you could see what we constantly deal with, you would slap yourself across the face and make changes in your life. If you were to let the stuff we see in the hospital dictate your view of aging and retirement, then you would have nothing to look forward to other than disability, sickness, and poor quality of life.

But then I remind myself that in the hospital setting, we rarely see healthy people. Our patients are almost never lean and muscular. That's because healthy people do not need hospitals unless something unpreventable happens, like a car accident. The healthy choices we make in life build up a defense against sickness, disease, and disability, and in turn we earn a comfortable aging experience and an enjoyable retirement.

On the other hand, the unhealthy choices we make in youth and middle age do not disappear, even though we cannot see the effects at the time. Every negative choice is painted inside your body's canvas. You might call it your grand masterpiece. This piece of art is your body, and every cell in it reflects the roadmap of where you have been and what you have done. Your life and all the decisions, actions, and behaviors you experience eventually erupt publicly for all to see, portrayed in a glorious explosion in the aging years. The negative choices in life stack up on each other, eventually moving from the inside to the outside, at which point they can no longer be ignored.

"We reap what we sow" is a fact, just as death is inevitable.

For two decades, I've worked with thousands of patients ranging from the young to the geriatric. Based on these years of experience, I have noted obvious correlations and predicaments that most repeating and recurrent patients share. If left unchecked, these observable trends in humanity may lead to poor quality of life and dependency on doctors, therapists, and nurses in the hospital setting. Eliminating these trends and traits in your life can prevent you from earning a poor quality of life and making the hospital your second home.

- Most of the people I encounter in the hospital have a life history absent of weight training and cardiovascular exercise.
- Most of the people are overweight, obese, or morbidly obese.
- Most of the people smoke or have smoked, drank or drink alcohol in excess, did or do drugs, and overeat or undereat.
- Most of the people are sedentary, don't exercise or weight train, and don't want to.
- Most of the people eat hyperpalatable, calorie-dense, high-fat, high-carb unhealthy food and don't want to stop. They don't want to hear how their diet is affecting their health and instead choose to live with the consequences.
- Most of the people have made constant unhealthy decision after unhealthy decision. Their body is a public display, their grand masterpiece revealing the decisions in their lifetime thus far.
- Most of the people are living in a body riddled with the negative side effects caused by a lifelong chain of choosing the heavy-handed unhealthy choices.
- Most of the people are sick, diseased, disabled, and impaired at baseline and are now dealing with a new illness, trauma, or ailment. In other words, the negative choices in life have converged into a storm to destroy them.
- Most of the people are on an accelerated path to mortality, or death before their time.
- Most of the people are drowning in their bad decisions, their storm, and need doctors, pharmacists, nurses, therapists, and

the many other members of the healthcare team to help them out of the storm and move on in life.

- Most of the people are living in regret . . . regret of not choosing health over pleasure.
- Most of the people are reaching out for help because they cannot do it on their own.
- Most of the people are just like you and me . . .
- Most of the people have dreams and wishes.
- Most of the people hope for healing, strengthening, and better health.
- Most of the people are lonely, sad, sometimes mad, and scared.
- Most of the people need compassion, caring, and leadership.
- Most of the people have family, friends, coworkers, and pets they are worried about.
- Most of the people desire change.
- Most of the people do not have the skills or knowledge to do it on their own. They need a health coach.

That is why I chose to write this and many other books. To provide resources for personal transformation. To be your health coach for under $30, compared to paying me or other trainers $50 to over $100 an hour. What a deal! This book is full of a professional's years of experience, knowledge, insight, risk-taking, and experimentation, saving you all the time it took to achieve by distilling it into mere hours of reading.

This book puts the power in your hands and gives you the recipe to make positive change happen for yourself. You can learn more life skills and resources for success in one book than you can in a college course. After all, if you want Bill Gates, Oprah Winfrey, Warren Buffet, Rachel Hollis, or Arnold Schwarzenegger to be your mentors, they wrote books for you. God also wrote a book for you to live a fulfilling life, the number-one-selling book in the history of mankind. Maybe you should read these books and harness the invaluable information that is waiting for you!

Healthy people do not need hospitals. Remember, over 70 percent of people in the US are overweight or obese, and this trend is only getting worse. In a hospital, it's more like four out of five people are in terrible physical shape. People who consistently make the heavy-handed healthy choices in life win a life of aging in place, or staying at home.

I chose a career as an OT to be able to use my knowledge and skills to help those drowning in their storm. Healthcare workers like me are lifeguards at the pool . . . the pool of life, you might say, and we are waiting in standby for the next drowning person. We jump in and provide whatever intervention is needed to save them from drowning, then they move on. The patient does not pay us a second thought, and we return to standby waiting for the next.

Before OT school, I was a certified personal trainer at Gold's Gym, powerlifter, martial artist, pincushion for nutritional manipulation and diet strategy, and winner of the Waterville/NCW fair's "tight fittin' jeans" contest two years in a row. I'm a certified fitness trainer through the International Sports Sciences Association (ISSA) and have been a National Physique Committee (NPC) competitive bodybuilder for over twenty years. I know what it takes to transform the human body to reach an optimal state of health.

Add to my knowledge on body transformation, dieting, and body-building, I have twenty years of hospital experience dealing with extreme cases of disease, disability, and aging. I witness firsthand what people are dealing with and observe the strong correlation between inflicted states and certain behaviors, past and present choices, and human physiology.

I have been working for years on designing programs and protocols and coaching to help people transform their lives—to earn *real* results. This is not placebo program bullshit. I yearn to make positive changes in the world one person at a time, one pound at a time, whether transforming lean mass or body fat, whether weight must be gained or lost—whatever your personal needs are.

Welcome to EXERLEAN.

EXERLEAN is the recipe for achieving and then living in a healthy body for life. The *EXER* pertains to cardiovascular exercise, weight training, aerobics, dance, sports, bodybuilding, and any other workload put on the body that makes it stronger, fit, and flexible. The *LEAN* refers to eating lean to be lean. A person must eat with a purpose. Just like a recipe for a cake must be followed for the best end product, we must follow the recipe—or algorithm—for making a lean, healthy, physically appealing body.

you + EXERLEAN = maximal health

EXERcising daily + eating LEAN
EXER + LEAN = EXERLEAN

Daily exercise plus healthy and restrictive nutrition—you cannot have one without the other.

This book hints at the *LEAN* and focuses on the *EXER*, in particular, weightlifting. First, we are going to go over the basics of exercise, weightlifting, and nutrition to establish the core body of knowledge you need to successfully transform your body. After we have established the knowledge core, we are going to get into the "meat" of the deal and focus heavily on Weight Chaining, or Chaining.

Weight Chaining is a designer workout protocol I have created that focuses on the anterior and posterior motor chains—that is, all the muscles in the front of your body and all the muscles in the back of your body, respectively. Working out in chains versus other formats improves functionality, promotes good posture against gravity, and provides a template that works out the whole body in just two workouts a week. We will go over preparation, tools, and everything else you need for your Weight Chaining agenda. We'll also review performance supplementation as well as workout routines, schedules, templates, and other bonus materials.

EXERLEAN provides all the necessary ingredients and steps for the recipe of physical awesomeness. Now, let's figure out how to bake your cake.

CHAPTER 1
THE GRAVITY OF RESISTANCE

There is one constant in our lives, a resistance that has no weakness. It's gravity, and the never-ending work our bodies go through to stand up against it. Gravity is on a relentless and infinite mission to pull our head down, curl our torso forward, drop us to the ground, and then pin us to the earth. We resist the pull of gravity from the moment we wake up in the morning until gravity wins and pulls us back into bed at night. During working hours, our posture is taxed. We fight to remain erect and in good posture. Nobody wants to become a hunchback or feel the pain of an unhealthy spine. So, we do a self-check periodically throughout the day and straighten up our posterior chain—those muscles on our backside, like our core and upper back—if we find ourselves slouching.

Nonetheless, the human body thrives in a gravity environment. The body needs this work to survive. For in the days we begin to lose the fight against gravity, we are likely dying or close to it.

A therapeutic session in the hospital setting involves introducing gravity back into a person's daily living routine. As an OT in the hospital, I first aim to help the patient get up off their back and at a minimum dangle on the edge of the hospital bed. This dose of gravity stimulates the respiratory, cardiovascular, and neuromuscular systems. Gravity becomes exercise for the person who is sick or disabled. If dangling at the edge of the bed is tolerated, the next aim is to stand, and if the patient can withstand gravity, they can begin to mobilize. Essentially, my number one goal as an OT is to help patients gain the strength and confidence to get out of the hospital bed and walk to the bathroom toilet rather than take a crap in the bed. If they can do this, we can move on to other daily mobility activities.

Life is a constant battle against gravity. The body will eventually succumb to the power of gravity at or near the end of life. There are actions we can take, however, to "kick the can down the road," you might say. To defer, deter, delay, and even prevent the negative sequence of events that gravity is destined to inflict on our bodies as we age. Aging of the human body is not the problem as much as the external forces against it. External forces become internal problems, like eating too much, eating unhealthy food, being sedentary, getting fat, smoking, getting drunk, and doing drugs.

We get out of bed, walk, climb, and rise against the forces of gravity in all waking moments of a day. We shower, dress, and prepare breakfast with gravity's constant tension pulling us to the earth's core. Gravity is the force that cumulatively wears us down at work, in rest, and at play. It is compounded with the mass of an object when moving, pushing, pulling, or fighting to lift it. Gravity can be a negative force in the context of an unhealthy or debilitated person. On the other hand, gravity is necessary to stay alive and thrive. The yin and the yang.

According to NASA, an astronaut will lose 22 percent of their blood volume after two to three days in outer space. The loss of blood is due to the absence of gravity, which on earth pulls the blood down to the feet and therefore decreases blood pressure in the brain. In outer space, there is no gravity to pull the blood down, therefore distributing blood volume evenly throughout the body. The increased volume in the upper body increases pressure on the brain in this zero-gravity environment. The brain senses the increased pressure and then signals the body to decrease its blood volume in order to lower the blood pressure in the upper body and head to normal levels. Coincidently, the heart begins to atrophy—basically waste away—due to the lightened workload, the lower extremities get skinny, and finally muscles atrophy and bone demineralizes.

Without gravity, the body does not need as much muscle or as dense a skeleton to survive. The muscles of the posterior chain, which hold us up against gravity on earth, can lose around 20 percent mass at a rate of 5 percent a week in a zero-gravity environment like space. An astronaut can lose 40 to 60 percent total bone mass at a rate of 1 percent a month while in space. Scientists know that exercise and resistance are key factors in maintaining muscle and bone mass in a zero-gravity environment.

Working out in the gym, taking a tai chi class, hiking or biking outdoors, and weight training exist only due to gravity. Without gravity, resistance would be a pointless endeavor. Without gravity, everything living and without life is weightless.

Resistance gives us purpose.

A purpose to fight, drive, and work against it in order to stay alive.

Without gravity, there is no resistance.

Without resistance, our bodies will deteriorate.

If your arm were extended and you released a rock from your hand, the rock would fall rapidly to the ground. Gravity is a relentless force against all things living and dead. Its strength is unwavering.

Humans use muscles encasing a bony skeleton that is built to power against the forces of gravity throughout the life span. This constant force pulling us to the core, or the center, of the earth will eventually win when we die. The focus for us all should not be on the inevitable end, however, but on the in-between. The time between conscious awareness and dementia. Crawling to walking to running, then crawling again. We should be moving to get shit done at a constant pace until old age fails us, cuts us off at the knees . . . or the hips, back, neck, or brain. If we strive at just one thing and one thing alone, we will maximize our productivity in all areas of life. That one thing is to fight like hell to stay master and controller over the force of gravity.

The mind alone has zero power against gravity's tension toward the earth's core. This is the job of your muscles, bones, and connective tissues. Thriving in life depends on our ability to hold our head up against gravity first, then our spine, shoulders, and arms. We can achieve the most laborious workloads when our lower body also pushes us away from the earth, moving us anywhere we choose to go.

The relentless fight against gravity—resistance—is our first and last fight for life.

The workload resistance provides is the necessary stimulation that provokes our bodies to strengthen, tone up, grow, and develop through-out life. We can enhance our bodies beyond gravity's effects by supple-menting with weight training or weightlifting. We can build a strong defense against gravity's pull by gaining rather than maintaining a strong posterior motor chain. With weight training, we can build our bodies into heavy-duty machines able to manipulate the environment around us. We can build up our metabolism and maximize the performance of our eating machine.

You control you and what actions you engage in. Weight training is a key tool in the war against gravity's ill effects and a death caused by obesity, sarcopenia, and ultimately failure to thrive.

CHAPTER 2

SEDENTARY TIME: FRENEMY OR ENEMY?

For every action, there is an equal and opposite reaction. This is Newton's third law of physics. The same principle can apply to any force—physical, mental, imaginary, or unknown. For every positive force, there is an equally negative one. The opposite force of gravity is antigravity. For every grand idea, plan, or passion of work, there is a counter-resistance equal to or less than the idea, plan, or passion, attempting to disrupt and sabotage it. For work, the foe or counterforce is sedentary behavior, a mindset that dwells in doing nothing. It's the opposite mindset of a worker bee to the hive and a productive asset to society.

My point is, every person has the power to fight those negative forces and accomplish anything they can imagine by taking action on it. Nothing different will result if they don't.

We all make decisions throughout the day for every day of our lives. Each decision has multiple choices we can execute. Each choice leads to a unique outcome. For every choice we make, there exists a benefit and a cost. The cost is the loss of what could have been, and the benefit is whatever outcome is achieved. The cost-benefit analysis (CBA) is a formula used in economics to help determine the heavy-handed beneficial choice of a decision. In my book *EXERLEAN*'s discussion on Bodinomics, or the economy of the human body, I advise readers to use the cost-benefit analysis to help make decisions on what and when to eat, drink, exercise, rest, and do everything else in our life mission to transform our body, mind, and soul toward peak health and maximal quality of life.

Sedentary time is not necessarily your enemy, but it is that of a friend-enemy . . . a frenemy. We hear so much negativity about *sedentary behavior*, but this must not be confused with *sedentary time*. Sedentary time can be your friend. Sedentary behavior causes the death of all things creative, productive, and physical. Sedentary time describes an action, purposefully doing nothing. Sedentary behavior describes a mindset, a personality expression drunk in laziness and lack of drive. Sedentary time is relaxing, restful, thoughtful, healing, and rewarding. There are many health benefits for taking time for moments of gratitude, reflection, meditation, relaxation, deep breathing, and sleep.

The body needs rest, but just enough. Too much rest will kill you. Restful time is not the same as laziness or indolence, which describe sedentary behavior. Let's take a look now at the best way to combat our sedentary lifestyles in our journey toward lifelong health.

CHAPTER 3
THE BENEFITS OF EXERCISE

You have probably heard a million times that exercise benefits you, but maybe you dismiss it. Many people do not fully understand exactly what exercise does to their own body because they do not exercise. Until you *feel* the benefits of exercise, you cannot fully *understand* the benefits. When you see your body composition changing for the better, and when you experience how great you feel after exercising, the reality of the benefits of exercise is pasted onto your physique, in your thoughts, and into how you feel.

Exercise leads to increased muscle tone, thermogenesis (metabolism) of body fat, and improved heart, lung, and circulatory function. The benefits of exercise are felt, seen, and realized in the flesh. Exercise is a natural phenomenon that changes the body within the first seconds of participation.

Your behavior and all the millions of beneficial, costly decisions you make in your life compose the canvas of your body. The costs of sedentary behavior and overeating lead to body fat being painted all over the canvas. You can feel and see the results of sedentary behavior—and likewise, your active behavior. What painting do you want to see? That of exercise or that of sedentary behavior? You decide, then engage in that behavior and reap the fruits of your choice. Don't take this decision lightly. One path leads to a healthy body, productivity, and longevity. The other, to disability, obesity, and early mortality. It's a near guarantee. We reap what we sow carries on through every cell in our body from birth to death, to the proliferation of new cells and the death of old cells, and so on.

When we exercise, our body goes through a monumental and stimulating metamorphosis. The first thing that happens with exercise is the resistance to gravity, and with that, our heart starts beating a bit faster. Resisting gravity is body weight exercise, albeit lower threshold and nothing compared to weightlifting; nonetheless, it's much better than lying still. While we're standing, our chest begins to rise and fall from head to toe rather than sternum to spine. As we get up and mobilize, blood circulates at a higher rate and blood pressure rises, awakening the distal tissues in the body (those farthest from the center). As exercise is initiated, whether hiking a mountain or using an elliptical trainer, our body then heats up and begins the thermogenic (i.e., heat-producing) process of metabolism.

We get a light amount of exercise by engaging in self-care and other *activities of daily living* (ADL). ADL involve things like gathering clothing and getting dressed, toilet transfer and toileting, bathing, grooming, and hygiene. *Instrumental activities of daily living* (IADL) are necessary work, like doing the laundry, cleaning the house, washing the dishes, cooking dinner, mowing the lawn, and driving the kids to school. ADLs and IADLs are light exercise compared to sleeping in bed. In fact, by enhancing your way of engaging in ADL and IADL, such as changing the variables and speed, you can further increase the exercise benefits.

For example, while engaging in ADL and IADL, move faster. I call the process *hyperactive ADL*. Move with haste while getting out of bed and walking to the bathroom, then getting dressed and showering. By moving faster, you increase your heart rate, which in turn increases your fat-burning metabolism. Same goes with IADL, but it provides even more of an exercise benefit because IADLs are generally more difficult, or of higher workload than ADL. Do your laundry like you're a dancing queen in a disco fever. Turn on your favorite music, crank up the volume, and let 'er rip. Vacuum, dust, and wash dishes with greater intensity, hyperactivity, and drive. This hyperactive behavior will give you enhanced benefit—and you haven't even actually exercised yet. This is also more efficient and productive in the grand scheme of things.

Walking is exercise compared to sitting in a chair, just like sitting in a chair is exercise compared to lying in bed. The farther your head is from the earth, the more you are resisting against the pull of gravity. The more you are resisting against gravity, the harder your muscles, heart, and lungs have to work. This is a good start, especially if you are beginning at a very low and sedentary baseline. One heavy-handed beneficially healthy choice at a time, you will win the war on body fat and lean muscle depravity.

Sedentary time can be purposeful and, as we said, sometimes a frenemy, such as sitting in a chair for your job. Although necessary, this time is not your friend. Too much sit time leads to negative health, disease, obesity, and poor quality of life in your aging years.

For those working a desk job, you can begin the fight on obesity and sedentary death by getting up and moving as often as possible. Break up all that sedentary time by resisting gravity, moving hyper-actively, and getting your heart beating faster. Engage your muscles. Every fifteen-minute break, hit the stairwell, front-entry steps, or uneven outdoor terrain. On your lunch break, go for a hyperactive walk and reflect on the positives in your life, listen to an audiobook, or visit with a cowalker. Get creative and pursue a better outcome for your physical and mental health. Trust me, your life depends on it. You will feel something positive, a reward of some sort the first time you do this. Then keep doing it over and over again until you can't think of doing anything else. This is how you develop a habit.

There are a few other things you can do at that desk job to get moving, like pedaling on a portable floor cycle, doing intermittent body weight sit-to-stands, or doing squats out of your chair. Stretch often. Ask your employer if you can have a standing desk so you can balance your sit time with time spent resisting gravity in the standing position. The benefits of exercise are key to attaining and then harnessing a life of health, wellness, and happiness.

Beyond the first steps of replacing as much sedentary time as possible with beneficial hyperactive, body weight activity and resistance to gravity, we can start a routine exercise program.

Exercise is when you engage the body in an activity that takes it out of its resting state. As your body starts working, physiologic reactions take place: your heart rate goes up, your blood circulates faster and is delivered to all areas of your body, your brain's alertness increases, and every cell in your body prepares for metabolism.

Metabolism is when your body changes food or stored energy like body fat into energy for work, measured in calories, to fuel the activity at hand. The harder the workload or resistance of the activity, the higher the demand to convert food or stored energy into fuel for work, play, or whatever you are exerting for. The harder the work, the more calories for fuel are needed.

Cardiovascular exercise, or cardio, increases the heart rate enough to trigger a release of endorphins, metabolism of calories, and thermogenesis of body fat. Cardio requires increased oxygen, meaning it is *aerobic*.

These types of activities include jogging, running, and spending time on a treadmill, elliptical, or stair mill. Weightlifting, on the other hand, is mostly considered an *anaerobic* activity, or without oxygen. Weightlifting puts a higher degree of stress on your muscle fibers and joints, maxing out your muscle use and harnessing the benefits of anabolism. Anabolism is a state of reactions that lead to growth, repair, and replacement of your body's cells.

Cardio should be a daily activity, whereas weight training requires longer rest periods between bouts to allow for maximal healing and recovery of damaged muscle tissue, a natural consequence of weightlifting.

Cardio is healthy for your heart, lungs, skin, brain, and other organs, as well as your eyes, nerves, digestion, and mind. Weight training stimulates the core, strengthens you, and prepares you for the workloads in your life. The perfect exercise scenario is a routine of cardio and weight training to ultimately prevent disease, disability, and early sedentary death.

In a resting state, 20–25 percent of your body's capillaries (tiny blood vessels) are open and moving blood. In a state of exercise, 100 percent of your body's capillaries are open and transporting blood, delivering vital nutrients to all areas of your body. Exercise increases heart rate and stroke volume, thus elevating your overall cardiac output. *Cardiac output* is the combination of your heart rate per minute, stroke volume, and blood pressure.

Heart rate is the number of times your heart beats in a minute. Stroke volume is the amount of blood that passes through the heart in one beat. Blood pressure describes your blood supply flowing from high-pressure areas to low-pressure areas, or from your heart to the farthest areas of your body. The quality of nutrient delivery throughout your body depends on several factors, including cardiac output, blood volume, and how well the circulatory system functions. If a person has peripheral vascular disease (PVD), peripheral artery disease (PAD), or some other impairment of their veins and arteries that compromises their circulatory system, then nutrient delivery to the farthest reaches of their body will be impaired, too. New research shows that obesity may be a cause or increase likeliness of acquiring peripheral artery disease, which 6.8 million Americans age forty and over suffer from.

Exercise can help us prevent further pruning of our veins and arteries. It improves circulation by creating more supply branches of capillaries and venules (tiny veins) to deliver nutrients to the farthest reaches of the body. Research has proven over and over again that exercise benefits cardiac output, improving circulation and preventing heart and peripheral vascular disease.

When we start exercising, we begin to breathe deeper, and our respiratory rate increases to increase the oxygen supply to our body tissues and then transport and exhale the waste product carbon dioxide. The overall conditioning of our body determines how our heart and lungs will perform during work or exercise. Our healthstyle—the daily routine, habits, and behaviors that dictate our current and future health—determines our conditioning, and the better our conditioning, the more efficient our system is at delivering oxygen and picking up carbon dioxide throughout the body to dispose of.

A healthy or conditioned person will have a lower overall respiratory or breath rate per minute than a deconditioned person. That is why a deconditioned person will huff and puff during exercise, whereas many conditioned or healthy people will have an unnoticeable change in respiratory rate doing the exact same exercise. As you change your body from weight training, cardio, or hyperactive ADL, at some point you will notice that, thanks to your improved conditioning, your body will endure longer and more difficult sessions without huffing and puffing.

How our body handles the total of all chemical changes within it results in either an anabolic or catabolic metabolism pathway.

Anabolism is a process that uses energy to join smaller molecules into larger ones. As we mentioned, an anabolic process incorporates growth, synthesis, replenishment, and repair of all tissues, hormones, and neurotransmitters in our body. Basically, anabolism leads to building or constructing our body and requires energy or fuel for the work. Anabolic metabolism should be simply thought of as a process of growth and repair of the body. Anabolism is the ultimate goal of all weightlifters, bodybuilders, and others who desire positive muscle mass transformation.

A state of growth is a good thing when it comes to repair and growth of lean body mass or muscle tissue, but it's a bad thing if there is an excess of calories. If not burned off during work or exercise, those extra calories are stored as body fat. During a strengthening or weight training program, it is wise to eat enough to repair and rebuild damaged muscle tissue yet prevent gaining excess body fat.

Catabolism is the opposite of anabolism. It is the destruction of the body, or breaking down larger molecules into smaller molecules. Anabolism uses nutrients or energy to create, whereas catabolism tears down the body to release energy. The energy derived from catabolism is used to facilitate anabolic reactions.

To keep it simple, a catabolic reaction is a breakdown or destruction of our body tissues and a process that releases energy or fuel for our body to use. The breakdown of skeletal muscle and the destruction of body fat are both catabolic. Think of catabolism as cannibalism, because a catabolic pathway in our body is in a way eating ourselves alive. I want you to strive to put your body into a state of metabolizing body fat, glycogen (stored sugar in muscle tissue), and food for fuel—*not* metabolizing your muscles!

This book is about gaining muscle mass, not losing it!

Lean muscle tissue does all the work. It is a productive asset unlike body fat, which is a total burden. Excess body fat has no benefit unless you are starving and need it for food or you live in a freezing environment, which are both lame excuses in an era where it is easy to get food, buy a warm coat, heat a house, or move to a warmer climate.

Did you know that you burn more calories the more muscle mass you have? Muscles burn calories just by existing. The more muscle tissue you have, the more calories you burn at rest than at work. Think about it. Muscles need energy just to live. Body fat just sits there and requires nothing. Gives nothing. People with extra body fat await a calorie deficit like a bear preparing for hibernation. Except they aren't hibernating!

Your resting metabolic rate is based on the amount of lean skeletal muscle you have; therefore, it makes sense that you should prioritize increasing muscle mass over burning body fat. Increasing muscle mass will help you succeed in your transformation through improving strength, increasing power, and boosting resting metabolic rate. Plus, fat burning is easier the more lean muscle you have.

As mentioned, exercise triggers endorphin release, which results in an elated mental state, an acute increase in cognitive awareness, and an overall positive sense of well-being. Wow! Doesn't that sound like something you want? Hell, yeah! Endorphins are the good-vibe hormones predominantly released into the bloodstream to treat pain and stress in our body. Endorphins react with the opiate receptors in our brain just like narcotic painkillers, alcohol, cocaine, and amphetamines do.

Naturally occurring endorphins are healthy. Endorphins from taking narcotics, cocaine, and amphetamines are not. In fact, prescription painkiller overdosing linked to "unintentional death" is now the number one preventable cause of death in the US. Cocaine and amphetamines are illegal and highly addictive drugs that destroy many people's lives. Alcohol is an over-the-counter beverage with obvious benefits but negative outcomes depending on the amount consumed and whether you abuse it or are addicted. All these substances cause an endorphin release into the bloodstream and create positive mood-altering effects, habit, and addiction. Since exercise also releases endorphins, it should be the number one weapon in the treatment plan to overcome these addictions. For your EXERLEAN Chaining endeavors, we will stick with getting our endorphins from exercise!

The endorphin release during exercise is long lasting. It will help you maintain a positive mood and help you feel energized and ready to tackle the world. Because of this, it is beneficial to get in your cardiovascular exercise first thing in the morning. Talk about getting a good start to the day and your foot out the door on a positive note.

Exercise promotes a ready state in all your body cells and your mind. This ready state boosts your mental health, helping you manage stress, pain, and depression and improving your self-confidence, mood, and overall mental state. The activation of all your cells also jacks your metabolic state and helps burn off calories and body fat for the remainder of the day. Another sustaining benefit of exercise and weight training includes improved hormone modulation.

Exercise is natural and within our control. Exercising daily can help people prevent and manage type 2 diabetes, reduce risks of some cancers, improve overall longevity, maintain and improve sexual function, improve sleep quality, quit smoking, strengthen bones, strengthen muscles, improve balance, and decrease the risk of falling. Exercise is one of the most natural and healthiest treatments for obesity, other diseases, and many disabilities. That's why it should always be considered the first medicine for treating and even curing obesity.

CHAPTER 4

THE BENEFITS OF WEIGHT TRAINING

L ifting weights leads to stronger, bigger, and toned muscles. Toned and ready to complete the physical challenging work in your life. Remember this: muscle mass—not bones or fat—is the only producer of physical work, namely in the forms of labor, play, ADL, IADL, and manipulation of our external environment, such as picking up and holding a baby, adjusting the sink faucet, moving a piece of furniture, or turning dirt in the garden. You arrange, adapt, or remodel the environment with the force of your muscles.

Bones support your muscles and need to be solid, but they don't do the work. Neither does body fat, which only weighs you down, adds unnecessary and unproductive work to your muscles, and creates a barrier between you and your skin. Too much body fat in front, and you can't see or even reach below your waist. This can be a big problem for men when it comes to urinating and an embarrassment for women with the obstruction of an abdominal pannus, a massive fat fold above the genitalia that drapes over the groin. Worse yet, massive truncal (trunk), hip, and buttocks fat leads to the inability to reach and wipe the ass after taking a dump. I've seen this firsthand hundreds of times, and it's a tragedy.

Muscle has no negative consequences, unless there is such a thing as *being too strong . . . having too high a metabolism . . . looking too damn sexy . . .* or *living longer*!

I'll take all that good stuff . . . wouldn't you?

Muscles are the ticket to freedom in many aspects of life. Freedom to eat more and not worry as much about getting fatter. Freedom to lift heavy stuff and move it around. Freedom to remain independent with self-care, ADL, and functional mobility. Freedom from dependency on others in your aging and retirement years.

I mentioned in the last chapter that the more lean muscle mass you have, the more calories you burn and the less chance you have of storing calories as body fat, even in a resting state. I hinted that muscle mass is the ultimate weapon against obesity. Think about it. When people want to lose weight, they cut calories and start exercising. Maybe the focus shouldn't be so much on cutting calories but on changing the calorie sources. Maybe the focus shouldn't be on cardio but on weight training and adding more muscle mass to raise our metabolic level, thus increasing our potential for metabolizing body fat, otherwise known as thermogenesis.

Bones do not burn body fat. Body fat does not burn body fat. Our organs use minimal body fat for energy, and muscles are responsible for burning the remaining fat the body doesn't need. The food we eat, glycogen, and body fat are the fuel for work, and muscles are the engine in the car. The bigger the motor, the more fuel is burned; therefore, bigger muscles burn more fat.

The more muscle you have, the more work you can accomplish. The person with the most muscle wins the most freedom tickets in the journey of life. Better sex ticket. Improved stamina and libido ticket. Muscle mass is the ticket to the fountain of youth. Everything in the body is better with as much muscle and as little body fat as naturally possible. *Naturally*, meaning without drugs and with daily consumption of high-quality protein and routine maximal weight training. With time, patience, and perseverance, this is the formula to acquire your best lean and muscular you.

This book is about improving your lean muscle mass. In particular, about unraveling the secrets to Weight Chaining or EXERLEAN Chaining, a designer weight training program. I could have just jumped right into chaining and focused solely on it, but you need to understand the physiology, science, and methods behind it to absorb it. Remember, the majority of us are overweight or obese, lacking sufficient muscle mass, and heading for a poor quality of life in our aging years. Being obese in our aging or retirement years exponentially raises our likelihood of becoming disabled, diseased, or dead before our natural genetic set point. This coming from the perspective that we are not born obese but eat ourselves into obesity. Much the same as smoking will lead to an early demise and poor quality of life much earlier than for someone who never smoked at all. Smoking is preventable, and so is obesity. The two exist because of choices people make in their daily lives.

We have come to a place in society where we are inpatient and want answers right now! It has become easy to skip the foundation of an exercise program and jump into it without following the instructions. We as a culture in most of the civilized world have become impatient and ungrateful for the work, for the study, and for building the foundation of success. Most of our foundations are built with straw, then the foundation is blown away and we crash and burn. Without the foundational understanding of human physiology, nutrition science, the benefits of exercise, and weight training, you will be building a house without the blueprint. You will not reach your goals this way. To be successful, you need to follow the instructions precisely. You need to learn the ways of winners, lay the foundation of knowledge brick by brick, and have a detailed blueprint to get the end results you want. The first sections of this book are exactly that—the foundation for success in your weight training endeavors.

When I decided to share my designer weightlifting protocol with the world, I knew that the best delivery would be through a book. So, on top of my full-time job and busy family life, I wrote from 3:00 a.m. to 5:00 a.m. every day until I finished it.

I chose to do the work.

I chose to give you everything you need to fully grasp the situation at hand.

For you to take this information and turn it into something life changing.

To give you the blueprint, the keys to the car, the roadmap so that you can initiate and conquer Weight Chaining.

When you are done reading, you will have built your foundation for a successful transformation that will last your lifetime.

So, What Exactly Is Weight Training?

The concept is simple. Pick shit up and put it back down. BOOM! That is weight training, otherwise referred to as weightlifting. It's lifting, pushing, or pulling up something that has weight. Whatever muscle or muscle group is doing the lifting, the work, is getting trained. The more a muscle or muscle group is trained, the greater the damage to muscle fibers. This results in a healing response that makes the muscles stronger, bigger, and better. You'll be ready to repeat the process and tackle the work again with less difficulty in each subsequent session.

When you use your muscles, your brain acknowledges the use, puts the information in its memory banks, and then responds to build them bigger and better. When your body is repeatedly bombarded with heavier than familiar workloads, it will adapt by increasing the size of the muscular system to compensate. If you don't use your muscles, your brain senses that the least amount of muscle tissue is needed to maintain homeostasis at the sedentary level; therefore, your body will eat its own muscles. This is catabolism—your brain cannibalizes your body, eating its muscle tissue down to the level needed for the average workload put on the body.

"Use it or lose it" runs true.

This is just nature running its course. The body seeks balance—always. In this case, a balance of necessary muscle mass to complete the average daily workload put on the body. It only needs enough body fat to maintain thermoregulation—that is, to regulate body heat—and supply energy for work. The same concept applies to bone density and strength. The body will only develop the skeletal system to the average daily needs of the human body.

Weight training done correctly and enough to make your body consistently uncomfortable will result in it adapting to the uncomfortable workload by growing. That is the name of the game. Lift heavy stuff repeatedly and routinely, never stopping until the game of life is over.

The goal of weight training is to achieve results, specifically:

1. To prevent muscle wasting
2. To increase strength and power
3. To increase muscle size
4. To maximize physical defense against predators, both human and nonhuman

5. To increase fight-or-flight potential
6. To acquire the physical means to deliver maximal offense against a bully, thug, robber, rapist, murderer, or other assailant
7. To maximize metabolism
8. To prevent disease and disability
9. To improve heart and circulation health
10. To improve respiration and lung health
11. To improve digestive health
12. To maintain good posture and resistance to gravity for life
13. To maximize balance, equilibrium, and righting reactions (i.e., remaining stable when changing from an upright position) toward external forces
14. To maintain the ability to get out of bed, stand up from a toilet, climb stairs, and self-care
15. To maximize libido, stamina, and sex—to become a sex machine

As humans, most of us love, enjoy sex, fight, protect, defend, nurture, and yearn for better health. If weight training will make all this better, then lift the heck out of anything and everything!

Knowing the positive results of weight training, why wouldn't everyone strive to get in the habit of routine lifting? Well, bad habits have taken the place of good habits, or good habits never existed, and it's up to the individual to make a change.

If you're not in a routine of exercise and weight training, you need only decide to exchange sedentary time with active time. It is a mindset change to improve your health and wellness at all costs. In most cases, the costs are your TV, smartphone, iPad, computer, internet, and other media. You can live without all these obstacles. You cannot live and thrive without exercise and weight training. Aging, obesity, and the negative effects of a sedentary lifestyle will likely lead to disease, disability, shitty quality of life in retirement, and possibly early death. The costs of eliminating all sedentary time, habits, and behaviors far underweigh the heavy-handed benefits of exercise, weight training, and restrictive eating.

There are many different ways to train with weights. This book will focus heavily on Weight Chaining. But before we dive into how to train, let's get some basic understanding about weight training.

Weight training begins with you, the resistance, and the location. The easiest place to access weights and exercise equipment is at a commercial gym. All you need is to pay the gym fees to become a member and then go in the door. Later on, we will go over what gear, clothing, and other gym essentials like your EXERBAG and EXERTOOLS will improve your gym experience.

Another fantastic location is in your home, that is, your home gym. If you build it, you will go. Speaking from experience, a home gym is an invaluable asset for working parents, businesspeople, or anyone else strapped for time. Having your gym at home allows you to get your exercise and weight training in at your convenience and to work around the day. The ultimate scenario is to have a home gym and a commercial gym membership to work out at home when the schedule is tight and make time to go to a commercial gym when possible, since a commercial gym has easy access to more and better equipment.

A home gym can be put together with used gym equipment found on Craigslist, eBay, Facebook Marketplace, or another outlet. If you are renting your home, it may be a bad idea to invest in a home gym because when you move, you will have to move it too. If you're renting,

I recommend a good elliptical trainer so you can engage in cardio first thing every morning. This will kick off your day on a great note. Then for weight training, get a membership at the best gym at a convenient location. If you own your home and plan to live there long term, then I recommend investing in a top-quality home gymnasium. Dedicate an area of your home to your health, whether it be the garage, a shop, the basement, or somewhere else.

The costs of a gym membership and home gym equipment is nothing compared to the negative benefits and costs of a lifetime of sedentary behavior and the shitstorm of diseases, disability, and poor quality of life to follow. Your life is what you make it. All thoughts, ideas, and dreams become reality if you take action, do the work, and focus on achieving the goal, the vision in your mind.

You can lift weights in any format you invent, plan, or follow. There are a gazillion different workout protocols, programs, formats, and plans, and they all work in varying degrees depending on your goals. I recommend a program that focuses on the principles of bodybuilding and strength gains. You want to maximize your muscle mass to both maximize your resting metabolic rate and become as strong as possible.

If you are new to weight training, then I recommend following my Weight Chaining program, starting with phase one. If you are a seasoned weightlifter, athlete, or bodybuilder looking to change things up with a new weight training protocol, then this is what you've been looking for.

When we get to the whole Weight Chaining program. I have included workout plans, format, exercise protocols, and many ways you can adapt or modify chaining to fit your desires. It is not necessary, but it may benefit you to hire a personal trainer for the first month to help you go through and learn the correct body mechanics, speed, range of motion, and form for all the weightlifting exercises in the program. This will ensure you master the foundational skills that will lead you to successful outcomes. Make it clear to the personal trainer that you are not hiring them for their own training regimen, ideas, or interests. At least not at this time. You are hiring them to help you master the EXERLEAN Weight Chaining protocol to promote extension (muscles extending and straightening) over flexion (muscles bending) and become master and commander of your body against the force of gravity.

Weight training damages the body, and then the body responds by healing itself to an even better condition to prepare itself for the next bout of work. The healing process requires the right nutrition. Although this book is not a nutrition book, you do need acquire a basic understanding of nutrition's role in muscle damage recovery. So, let's breeze through the nutrition basics and what is needed to help you recover from your brutal weightlifting sessions.

RESOURCES

1. *Delusions of Crowds*, by William J. Bernstein. (Feb 23, 2021). Atlantic Monthly Press.
2. https://www.vice.com/en/article/evkmkz/how-gross-is-it-if-i-cant-wipe-my-butt-after-pooping
3. https://www.tonyrobbins.com/leadership-impact/the-secret-to-living-is-giving/
4. https://www.health.com/condition/stress/ways-debt-is-bad-for-your-health
5. Jacobson BH, Boolani A, Dunklee G, Shepardson A, Acharya H. Effect of prescribed sleep surfaces on back pain and sleep quality in patients diagnosed with low back and shoulder pain. Appl Ergon. 2010 Dec;42(1):91-7. doi: 10.1016/j.apergo.2010.05.004. Epub 2010 Jun 26. PMID: 20579971.
6. https://www.takingcharge.csh.umn.edu/prayer
7. *Think and Grow Rich*, by Napolean Hill. (1937). The Ralston Society.
8. *The Strangest Secret*, by Earl Nightingale. (1956). Nightingale-McHugh Company
9. *Collected Works of Abraham Lincoln*. Volume 2. Lincoln, Abraham, 1809-1865; https://quod.lib.umich.edu/l/lincoln/lincoln2/1:346?rgn=div1;view=fulltext

REFERENCES

All things in moderation? threshold effects in adolescent extracurricular participation intensity and behavioral problems - pubmed. (2019). PubMed. https://pubmed.ncbi.nlm.nih.gov/30604445/

Balance and moderation quotes. (2021). https://www.quotegarden.com/golden-mean.html

Bernstein, L. R., Pharm.D. (2020). *Time to quit: covid-19 is another reason to stop smoking.* https://www.costcoconnection.com/connection/202012/MobilePagedArticle.action?articleId=1641689

Boldrini, M., MD, PhD., Canoll, P. D., MD, PhD., & Klein, R. S., MD, PhD. (2021). *How covid-19 affects the brain.* JAMA network. https://jamanetwork.com/journals/jamapsychiatry/fullarticle/2778090

Changes in back pain, sleep quality, and perceived stress after introduction of new bedding systems. (2008). PubMed Central (PMC). https://www.ncbi.nlm.nih.gov/pmc/articles/PMC2697581/

Digging a vegetarian diet. (2017, June 27). NIH News in Health. https://newsinhealth.nih.gov/2012/07/digging-vegetarian-diet

Everything in moderation--dietary diversity and quality, central obesity and risk of diabetes - pubmed. (2015). PubMed. https://pubmed.ncbi. nlm.nih.gov/26517708/

Feeling out of joint. (2017, December 5). NIH News in Health. https:// newsinhealth.nih.gov/special-issues/seniors/feeling-out-joint

Fixing flawed body parts. (2017, May 9). NIH News in Health. https:// newsinhealth.nih.gov/2015/02/fixing-flawed-body-parts

G52. (2006). *Mht_spirituality.indd* [PDF]. https://www.mentalhealth. org.uk/sites/default/files/impact-spirituality.pdf

Good sleep for good health. (2021, March 29). NIH News in Health. https://newsinhealth.nih.gov/2021/04/good-sleep-good-health

How do people define moderation? - pubmed. (2016). PubMed. https:// pubmed.ncbi.nlm.nih.gov/26964691/

How mindfulness training can boost your immune system. (2018, January 25). Cleveland Clinic. https://health.cleve-landclinic.org/how-mindfulness-training-can-help-you-achieve-immunologic-health/

Is "everything in moderation" terrible advice? (2021, March 9). Nutritional Weight and Wellness. https://www.weightandwellness.com/resources/ articles-and-videos/everything-moderation-terrible-advice/

Managing asthma. (2017, May 15). NIH News in Health. https://news-inhealth.nih.gov/2014/06/managing-asthma

Managing pain. (2018, September 24). NIH News in Health. https://newsinhealth.nih.gov/2018/10/managing-pain

Mcn | medical consultants network: the consequences of not working. (n.d.). MCN | Medical Consultants Network. https://mcn.com/mcntalk/page/19/

Mindfulness meditation: A research-proven way to reduce stress. (2019). https://www.apa.org. https://www.apa.org/topics/mindfulness/meditation

Mindfulness meditation and the immune system: A systematic review of randomized controlled trials. (2016). PubMed Central (PMC). https://www.ncbi.nlm.nih.gov/pmc/articles/PMC4940234/

Mouth microbes. (2019, April 30). NIH News in Health. https://news-inhealth.nih.gov/2019/05/mouth-microbes

One day of employment a week is all we need for mental health benefits. (2019). ScienceDaily. https://www.sciencedaily.com/releases/2019/06/190618192030.htm

Personalized exercise? (2020, June 30). NIH News in Health. https://newsinhealth.nih.gov/2020/07/personalized-exercise

Please stop saying "everything in moderation" - the whole30® program. (2013, August 12). The Whole30® Program. https://whole30. com/moderation/

Prayer and healing. a case study - pubmed. (1997). PubMed. https:// pubmed.ncbi.nlm.nih.gov/9287623/

Prayer and healing: A medical and scientific perspective on randomized controlled trials. (2009). PubMed Central (PMC). https://www.ncbi. nlm.nih.gov/pmc/articles/PMC2802370/

Researchers working from home: Benefits and challenges. (2021). PubMed Central (PMC). https://www.ncbi.nlm.nih.gov/pmc/ articles/PMC7993618/

Risks to healthcare organizations and staff who manage obese (bariatric) patients and use of obesity data to mitigate risks: A literature review. (2021). PubMed Central (PMC). https://www.ncbi.nlm.nih.gov/ pmc/articles/PMC7954428/

Role of sleep and sleep loss in hormonal release and metabolism - pubmed. (2009). PubMed. https://pubmed.ncbi.nlm.nih.gov/19955752/

Seeing is believing: The power of visualization. (2009). Psychology Today. https://www.psychologytoday.com/us/blog/flourish/200912/ seeing-is-believing-the-power-visualization

7 health effects of working too much. (2017). Healthline. https://www. healthline.com/health/working-too-much-health-effects

Spiritual health and wellness. (2022). https://www.mit.edu/~rei/spir-immune.html

The benefits of slumber. (2017, May 31). NIH News in Health. https://newsinhealth.nih.gov/2013/04/benefits-slumber

The effect of long working hours and overtime on occupational health: A meta-analysis of evidence from 1998 to 2018. (2019). PubMed Central (PMC). https://www.ncbi.nlm.nih.gov/pmc/articles/PMC6617405/

The science of visualization: Maximizing your brain's potential during the recession. (2009, April 3). HuffPost. https://www.huffpost.com/entry/the-science-of-visualizat_b_171340

Therapeutic modalities – pm&r knowledgenow. (2016). https://now.aapmr.org/therapeutic-modalities/

Varga, L., Pharm.D. (2020). *When viruses collide.* For you health. https://www.costcoconnection.com/connection/202012/MobileP-agedArticle.action?articleId=1641692

Zrull, M. (2020). *Microsoft word - hynes and turner (2020) to post.docx* [PDF]. https://impulse.appstate.edu/sites/impulse.appstate.edu/files/Hynes and Turner (2020).pdf

www.ingramcontent.com/pod-product-compliance
Lightning Source LLC
Chambersburg PA
CBHW062115020426
42335CB00013B/976